How to Write a Paper

FOURTH EDITION

How to Write a Paper

FOURTH EDITION

Edited by

George M. Hall

St George's
University of London
London, UK

BMJ|Books

Blackwell
Publishing

© 1994 by BMJ Publishing Group
© 2008 by Blackwell Publishing

BMJ Books is an imprint of the BMJ Publishing Group Limited, used under licence

Blackwell Publishing, Inc., 350 Main Street, Malden, Massachusetts 02148-5020, USA

Blackwell Publishing Ltd, 9600 Garsington Road, Oxford OX4 2DQ, UK

Blackwell Publishing Asia Pty Ltd, 550 Swanston Street, Carlton, Victoria 3053, Australia

The right of the Author to be identified as the Author of this Work has been asserted in accordance with the Copyright, Designs and Patents Act 1988.

First published 1994 by BMJ
Second edition 1998
Third edition 2003
Fourth edition 2008

5   2010

Library of Congress Cataloging-in-Publication Data

How to write a paper / edited by George M. Hall.—4th ed.
    p. ; cm.
Includes bibliographical references and index.
ISBN 978-1-4051-6773-4 (alk. paper)
1. Medical writing.   I.   Hall, George M.   (George Martin)
[DNLM: 1. Writing. 2. Publishing.   WZ 345 H847 2008]
R119.H69 2008
808'.06661—dc22

                                                                2007036933

A catalogue record for this title is available from the British Library

Set by Charon Tec Ltd (A Macmillan Company), Chennai, India

Printed and bound in Singapore by Fabulous Printers Pte Ltd

Commissioning Editor: Mary Banks
Development Editor: Simone Dudziak
Production Controller: Rachel Edwards

For further information on Blackwell Publishing, visit our website:

http://www.blackwellpublishing.com

The publisher's policy is to use permanent paper from mills that operate a sustainable forestry policy, and which has been manufactured from pulp processed using acid-free and elementary chlorine-free practices. Furthermore, the publisher ensures that the text paper and cover board used have met acceptable environmental accreditation standards.

Contents

List of Contributors

Robert N. Allan
Editor, *Clinical Medicine*
Royal College of Physicians
London, UK
Formerly: Consultant Physician and
Gastroenterologist
University Hospital Birmingham
NHS Foundation Trust
Birmingham, UK

Craig Bingham
Publisher
Formerly: Communication
Development Manager
Australasian Medical
Publishing Company
Sydney, Australia

Margaret Cooter
Managing Technical Editor
BMJ Publishing Group
London, UK

Natalie Davies
Editorial Operations Manager
The Lancet
London, UK

Michael Doherty
Professor of Rheumatology
University of Nottingham
Nottingham, UK

Formerly: Editor, *Annals of the Rheumatic Diseases*

Gordon B. Drummond
Senior Lecturer
Department of Anaesthesia
Critical Care and Pain Medicine
University of Edinburgh
Edinburgh, UK
Formerly: Editor, *British Journal of Anaesthesia*

Michael J.G. Farthing
Vice Chancellor
University of Sussex
Falmer, UK
Formerly: Editor, *Gut*

Paul Glasziou
Director, Centre for Evidence-
Based Medicine
Department of Primary Health Care
University of Oxford
Oxford, UK
Editor, *Evidence-Based Medicine*

George M. Hall
Professor of Anaesthesia
St George's
University of London
London, UK
Formerly: Chairman, *British Journal of Anaesthesia*

Richard Horton
Editor-in-Chief/Publisher,
The Lancet
London, UK

Simon Howell
Senior Lecturer in Anaesthesia
University of Leeds
Leeds, UK
Editor, *British Journal of Anaesthesia*

Jennifer M. Hunter
Professor of Anaesthesia
Department of Anaesthesia
Clinical Sciences
University of Liverpool
Liverpool, UK
Formerly: Editor-in-chief, *British Journal of Anaesthesia*

Domhnall MacAuley
Editor, *Primary Care*
BMJ
London, UK

Fiona Moss CBE
Dean of Postgraduate Medicine
London Deanery
NHS London
London, UK

Liz Neilly
Medical Librarian
University of Leeds
Leeds, UK

Hans-Joachim Priebe
Professor of Anaesthesia
Department of Anaesthesia
University Hospital
Freiburg, Germany
Editorial Board, *British Journal of Anaesthesia*

Martin Neil Rossor
Professor of Clinical Neurology
Editor, *Journal of Neurology, Neurosurgery and Psychiatry*
Dementia Research Centre
London, UK

Richard Smith CBE
Chief Executive
UnitedHealth Europe
London, UK
Formerly: Editor, *BMJ*

Mark Ware
Director, Mark Ware Consulting
Bristol, UK

Alex Williamson
Publishing Director
BMJ and BMJ Journals
BMJ Group
London, UK

Preface to the Third Edition

The unexpected success of the first and second editions of this short book and the rapid progress in certain areas of publishing have necessitated a third edition. The original intention was that it would appeal primarily to authors for whom English was not their first language. Sales in the United Kingdom, however, show that it has met a local need. For the third edition, it is a pleasure to welcome Craig Bingham, Margaret Cooter, Natalie Davies, Simon Howell, Domhnall MacAuley, Harvey Marcovitch, Fiona Moss, Hans Joachim Priebe, and Leo van de Putte as new contributors. An additional chapter, 'Electronic submissions', has been added.

I am grateful to all authors for revising their chapters and, in particular, to Robert Allan, Michael Doherty, Gordon Drummond, Graham Smith, Richard Smith, Tony Wildsmith, and Alex Williamson for contributing to all three editions.

George M. Hall

Preface to the Fourth Edition

For the fourth edition, it is a pleasure to welcome Paul Glasziou, Jennie Hunter, Liz Neilly, Martin Rossor, and Mark Ware as new contributors. An additional chapter, 'Open access', has been added.

I am grateful to all the authors for revising their chapters and, in particular, to Robert Allan, Michael Doherty, Gordon Drummond, Richard Smith, and Alex Williamson for contributing to all four editions.

George M. Hall

Chapter 1 **Structure of a scientific paper**

George M. Hall

The research you have conducted is obviously of vital importance and must be read by the widest possible audience. It probably is safer to insult a colleague's spouse, family, and driving than the quality of his or her research. Fortunately, so many medical journals now exist that your chances of not having the work published somewhere are small. Nevertheless, the paper must be constructed in the approved manner and presented to the highest possible standards. Editors and assessors without doubt will look adversely on scruffy manuscripts – regardless of the quality of the science. All manuscripts are constructed in a similar manner, although some notable exceptions exist, like the format used by Nature. Such exceptions are unlikely to trouble you in the early stages of your research career.

The object of publishing a scientific paper is to provide a document that contains sufficient information to enable readers to:
• assess the observations you made;
• repeat the experiment if they wish;
• determine whether the conclusions drawn are justified by the data.
The basic structure of a paper is summarised by the acronym IMRAD, which stands for:

Introduction   (What question was asked?)
Methods   (How was it studied?)
Results   (What was found?)
And
Discussion   (What do the findings mean?)

The next four chapters of this book each deal with a specific section of a paper, so the sections will be described only in outline in this chapter.

Introduction

The introduction should be brief and must state clearly the question that you tried to answer in the study. To lead the reader to this point, it is necessary to review the relevant literature briefly.

Many junior authors find it difficult to write the introduction. The most common problem is the inability to state clearly what question was asked. This should not be a problem if the study was planned correctly – it is too late to rectify basic errors when attempting to write the paper. Nevertheless, some studies seem to develop a life of their own, and the original objectives can easily be forgotten. I find it useful to ask collaborators from time to time what question we hope to answer. If I do not receive a short clear sentence as an answer, then alarm bells ring.

The introduction must not include a review of the literature. Only cite those references that are essential to justify your proposed study. Three citations from different groups usually are enough to convince most assessors that some fact is 'well known' or 'well recognised', particularly if the studies are from different countries. Many research groups write the introduction to a paper before the work is started, but you must never ignore pertinent literature published while the study is in progress.

An example introduction might be:

> It is well known that middle-aged male runners have diffuse brain damage,[1–3] but whether this is present before they begin running or arises as a result of repeated cerebral contusions during exercise has not been established. In the present study, we examined cerebral function in a group of sedentary middle-aged men before and after a six month exercise programme. Cerebral function was assessed by …

Methods

This important part of the manuscript increasingly is neglected, and yet the methods section is the most common cause of absolute rejection of a paper. If the methods used to try to answer the question were inappropriate or flawed, then there is no salvation for the work. Chapter 3 contains useful advice about the design of the study and precision of measurement that should be considered when the work is planned – not after the work has been completed.

The main purposes of the methods section are to describe, and sometimes defend, the experimental design and to provide enough detail that a competent worker could repeat the study. The latter is particularly important when you are deciding how much to include in the text. If standard methods of measurement are used, appropriate references are all that is required. In many instances, 'modifications' of published methods are used, and it is these that cause difficulties for other workers. To ensure reproducible data, authors should:
- give complete details of any new methods used;
- give the precision of the measurements undertaken;
- sensibly use statistical analysis.

The use of statistics is not covered in this book. Input from a statistician should be sought at the planning stage of any study. Statisticians invariably are helpful, and they have contributed greatly to improving both the design and analysis of clinical investigations. They cannot be expected, however, to resurrect a badly designed study.

Results

The results section of a paper has two key features: there should be an overall description of the major findings of the study; and the data should be presented clearly and concisely.

You do not need to present every scrap of data that you have collected. A great temptation is to give all the results, particularly if they were difficult to obtain, but this section should contain only relevant, representative data. The statistical analysis of the results must be appropriate. The easy availability of statistical software packages has not encouraged young research workers to understand the principles involved. An assessor is only able to estimate the validity of the statistical tests used, so if your analysis is complicated or unusual, expect your paper to undergo appraisal by a statistician.

You must strive for clarity in the results section by avoiding unnecessary repetition of data in the text, figures, and tables. It is worthwhile stating briefly what you did not find, as this may stop other workers in the area undertaking unnecessary studies.

Discussion

The initial draft of the discussion is almost invariably too long. It is difficult not to write a long and detailed analysis of the literature that you know so well. A rough guide to the length of this section, however, is that it should not be more than one-third of the total length of the manuscript (Introduction + Methods + Results + Discussion). Ample scope often remains for further pruning.

Many beginners find this section of the paper difficult. It is possible to compose an adequate discussion around the points given in Box 1.1.

Box 1.1 Writing the discussion

- Summarise the major findings
- Discuss possible problems with the methods used
- Compare your results with previous work
- Discuss the clinical and scientific (if any) implications of your findings
- Suggest further work
- Produce a succinct conclusion

Common errors include repetition of data already given in the results section, a belief that the methods were beyond criticism, and preferential citing of previous work to suit the conclusions. Good assessors will seize upon such mistakes, so do not even contemplate trying to deceive them.

Although IMRAD describes the basic structure of a paper, other parts of a manuscript are important. The title, summary (or abstract), and list of authors are described in Chapter 6. It is salutary to remember that many people will read the title of the paper and some will read the summary, but very few will read the complete text. The title and summary of the paper are of great importance for indexing and abstracting purposes, as well as enticing readers to peruse the complete text. The use of appropriate references for a paper is described in Chapter 7; this section often is full of mistakes. A golden rule is to list only relevant, published references and to present them in a manner that is appropriate for the particular journal to which the article is being submitted. The citation of large numbers of references is an indicator of insecurity – not of scholarship. An authoritative author knows the important references that are appropriate to the study.

Before you start the first draft of the manuscript, carefully read the 'Instructions to authors' that every journal publishes, and prepare your paper accordingly. Some journals give detailed instructions, often annually, and these can be a valuable way of learning some of the basic rules. A grave mistake is to submit a paper to one journal in the style of another; this suggests that it has recently been rejected. At all stages of preparation of the paper, go back and check with the instructions to authors to make sure that your manuscript conforms. It seems very obvious, but if you wish to publish in the *European Annals of Andrology*, do not write your paper to conform with the *Swedish Journal of Androgen Research*. Read and re-read the instructions to authors.

Variations on the IMRAD system are sometimes necessary in specialised circumstances, such as a letter to the editor (Chapter 9), an abstract for presentation at a scientific meeting (Chapter 10), or a case report (Chapter 11). Nevertheless, a fundamental structure is the basis of all scientific papers.

Chapter 2 **Introductions**

Richard Smith

Introductions should be short and arresting and tell the reader why you have undertaken the study. This first sentence tells you almost everything I have to say and you could stop here. If you were reading a newspaper, you probably would – and that is why journalists writing a news story will try to give the essence of their story in the first line. An alternative technique used by journalists and authors is to begin with a sentence so arresting that the reader will be hooked and likely to stay for the whole piece.

I may mislead by beginning with these journalistic devices, but I want to return to them: scientific writing can usefully borrow from journalism. But let me begin with writing introductions for scientific papers.

Before beginning, answer the basic questions

Before sitting down to write an introduction you must have answered the basic questions that apply to any piece of writing:
- What do I have to say?
- Is it worth saying?
- What is the right format for the message?
- What is the audience for the message?
- What is the right journal for the message?

If you are unclear about the answers to these questions then your piece of writing – no matter whether it's a news story, a poem, or a scientific paper – is unlikely to succeed. As editor of the *British Medical Journal*, every day I saw papers where the authors had not answered these questions. Authors are often not clear about what they want to say. They start with some sort of idea and hope that the reader will have the wit to sort out what is important. The reader will not bother. Authors also regularly choose the wrong format – a scientific paper rather than a descriptive essay or a long paper rather than a short one. Not being clear about the audience is probably the commonest error and specialists regularly write for generalists in a way that is entirely inaccessible.

5

Another basic rule is to read the instructions to authors (or advice to contributors, as politically correct journals like the *BMJ* now call them) of the journal you are writing for. Too few authors do this, but there is little point in writing a 400 words introduction when the journal has a limit for the whole article of 600 words.

Tell readers why you have undertaken the study

The main job of the introduction is to tell readers why you have undertaken the study. If you set out to answer a question that really interested you, then you will have little difficulty. But if your main reason for undertaking the study was to have something to add to your curriculum vitae, it will show. The best questions may arise directly from clinical practice and, if that is the case, the introduction should say so:

> A patient was anaesthetised for an operation to repair his hernia and asked whether the fact that he used Ecstasy four nights a week would create difficulties. We were unable to find an answer in published medical reports and so designed a study to answer the question.

or

> Because of pressure to reduce night work for junior doctors we wondered if it would be safe to delay operating on patients with appendicitis until the morning after they were admitted.

If your audience is interested in the answer to these questions then they may well be tempted to read the paper and, if you have defined your audience and selected the right journal, they should be interested.

More commonly, you will be building on scientific work already published. It then becomes essential to make clear how your work adds importantly to what has gone before.

Clarify what your work adds

Editors will not want to publish – and readers will not want to read – studies that simply repeat what has been done several times before. Indeed, you should not be undertaking a study or writing a paper unless you are confident that it adds importantly to what has gone before. The introduction should not read:

> Several studies have shown that regular Ecstasy use creates anaesthetic difficulties,[1–7] and several others have shown that it does not.[8–14] We report two further patients, one of whom experienced problems and one of whom did not, and review the literature.

Rather it should read something like:

> Two previous studies have reported that regular Ecstasy use may give rise to respiratory problems during anaesthesia. These studies were small and uncontrolled, used only crude measurements of respiratory function, and did not follow up the patients. We report a larger, controlled study, with detailed measurements of respiratory function and two year follow up.

Usually, it is not so easy to make clear how your study is better than previous ones and this is where the temptation arises to give a detailed critique of everything that has ever gone before. You will be particularly tempted to do this because, if you are serious about your study, you will have spent hours in the library detecting and reading all the relevant literature. The very best introductions will include a systematic review of all the work that has gone before and a demonstration that new work is needed.

The move towards systematic reviews is one of the most important developments in science and scientific writing in the past 20 years [1]. We now understand that most reviews are highly selective in the evidence they adduce and often wrong in the conclusions they reach [2]. When undertaking a systematic review an author poses a clear question, gathers all relevant information (published in whatever language or unpublished), discards the scientifically weak material, synthesises the remaining information, and then draws a conclusion.

To undertake such a review is clearly a major task, but this ideally is what you should do before you begin a new study. You should then undertake the study only if the question cannot be answered and if your study will contribute importantly to producing an answer. You should include a brief account of the review in the introduction. Readers will then fully understand how your study fits with what has gone before and why it is important.

'In 2007 you should not worry that you cannot reach this high standard because the number of medical papers that have ever done so could probably be numbered on the fingers of one hand'. I wrote the same sentence in the first edition of this book only with the year as 1994. I then wrote in the first edition: 'But by the end of the millennium brief accounts of such reviews will, I hope, be routine in introductions'. I was – as always – wildly overoptimistic. Summaries of systematic reviews are still far from routine in introductions in scientific papers. Indeed, a paper presented at the *Third International Congress on Peer Review* in September 1997 showed that many randomised controlled trials published in the world's five major general medical journals failed to mention trials that had been done before on the same subject.

This means that authors are routinely flouting the Helsinki Declaration on research involving human subjects. The declaration states that such research should be based on a thorough knowledge of the scientific literature [3]. Repeating research that has already been satisfactorily done is poor practice. As the CONSORT statement on good practice in reporting clinical trials says: 'Some clinical trials have been shown to have been unnecessary because the question they addressed had been or could have been answered by a systematic review of the existing literature' [4,5].

In 2007 my advice on systematically reviewing previous reports remains a counsel of perfection, but it's still good advice. Perhaps you can be somebody who moves the scientific paper forward rather than somebody who just reaches the minimum standard for publication.

Another important and relevant advance since the first edition is that scientific journals almost all now have websites and publish synergistically on paper and on the Web [6,7]. This at last opens up the possibility of simultaneously being able to satisfy the needs of the reader–researcher, who wants lots of detail and data, and the needs of the reader–practitioner, who wants a straightforward message. The *BMJ*, for example, introduced a system it calls ELPS (electronic long, paper short) [8]. In this case, it is the editors who produce the shorter paper, although you will have to approve it before publication. In the context of introductions, this synergistic publishing might mean that a proper systematic review might be published on the Web while the paper version might include a short and simple summary. Usually, however, a full systematic review is probably best dealt with as a separate paper.

One interesting feature of revising a chapter 13 years after you wrote the first version is to reflect on how much scientific papers have changed. We might have expected that the appearance of the World Wide Web in the early 1990s would have changed everything. Space is no longer a problem. Video and sound can be added. Hyperlinks are easy. Full data – and the software used to manipulate them – could be included. But the overwhelming impression so far is that very little has changed [9]. In 2004 the *BMJ* published the 50-year results of the British doctors study [10], providing an opportunity to compare the paper with that giving the first set of results half a century ago [11]. Making the comparison I wrote: 'In the 50 years during which men have landed on the moon, computers and the Internet have appeared, television and cars have been transformed, the scientific article has changed hardly at all. Does this reflect the robustness of the form or a failure of imagination? I suspect the latter' [9].

My suspicion is that new technology will eventually lead to dramatic changes and that if I live to write this chapter again I may have to start completely afresh.

Following the best advice

An important development in medical writing in recent years has been the appearance of suggested structures for certain kinds of studies. These have appeared because of considerable evidence that many scientific reports do not include important information. There are guidelines for randomised controlled trials [4], systematic reviews [12], economic evaluations [13], and studies reporting tests of diagnostic methods [14]. More guidelines will follow and many journals, including the *BMJ*, require authors to conform to these standards. They will send back reports that do not conform. So authors need to be aware of these guidelines. The requirements for introductions are usually straightforward and not very different from the advice given in this chapter.

Keep it short

You must resist the temptation to impress readers by summarising everything that has gone before. They will be bored, not impressed, and will probably never make it through your study. Your introduction should not read:

> Archaeologists have hypothesised that a primitive version of Ecstasy may have been widely used in ancient Egypt. Canisters found in tombs of the pharaohs … Sociological evidence shows that Ecstasy is most commonly used by males aged 15 to 25 at parties held in aircraft hangars? The respiratory problems associated with Ecstasy may arise at the alveolar–capillary interface. Aardvark hypothesised in 1926 that problems might arise at this interface because of?

Nor should you write:

> Many studies have addressed the problem of Ecstasy and anaesthesia.[1–9]

With such a sentence you say almost nothing useful and you've promptly filled a whole page with references. You should choose references that are apposite, not simply to demonstrate that you've done a lot of reading.

It may often be difficult to make clear in a few words why your study is superior to previous ones, but you must convince editors and readers that it is better. Your introduction might read something like:

> Anaesthetists cannot be sure whether important complications may arise in patients who regularly use Ecstasy. Several case studies have described such problems.[1–4] Three cohort studies have been published, two of which found a high incidence of respiratory problem in regular

Ecstasy users. One of these studies was uncontrolled[5] and in the other the patients were poorly matched for age and smoking.[6] The study that did not find any problems included only six regular Ecstasy users and the chance of an important effect being missed (a type II error) was high.[7] We have undertaken a study of 50 regular Ecstasy users with controls matched for age, smoking status, and alcohol consumption.

A more detailed critique of the other studies can be left for the discussion. Even then, you should not give an exhaustive account of what has gone before but should concentrate on the best studies that are closest to yours. You will also then be able to compare the strengths and weaknesses of your study with the other studies, something that would be wholly out of place in the introduction.

Make sure that you are aware of earlier studies

I've already emphasised the importance of locating earlier studies. Before beginning a study, authors should seek the help of librarians in finding any earlier studies. Authors should also make personal contact with people who are experts in the subject and who may know of published studies that library searches do not find, unpublished studies, or studies currently under way. It's also a good idea to find the latest possible review on the subject and search the references and to look at the abstracts of meetings on the subject. We know that library searches often do not find relevant papers that have already been published, that many good studies remain unpublished (perhaps because they reach negative conclusions), and that studies take years to conduct and sometimes years to get into published reports.

Editors increasingly want to see evidence that authors have worked hard to make sure that they know of studies directly related to theirs. This is particularly important when editors' first reaction to a paper is 'Surely we know this already'. We regularly had this experience at the *BMJ* and we then looked especially hard to make sure that authors had put effort into finding what had gone before.

In a systematic review the search strategy clearly belongs in the methods section, but in an ordinary paper it belongs in the introduction, in as short a form as possible. Thus it might read:

A Medline search using 15 different key phrases, personal contact with five experts in the subject, and a personal search of five recent conferences on closely related subjects produced no previous studies of whether grandmothers suck eggs.

Be sure your readers are convinced of the importance of your question, but don't overdo it

If you have selected the right audience and a good study then you should not have to work hard to convince your readers of the importance of the question you are answering. One common mistake is to start repeating material that is in all the textbooks and that your readers will know. Thus, in a paper on whether vitamin D will prevent osteoporosis you do not need to explain osteoporosis and vitamin D to your readers. You might, however, want to give them a sense of the scale of the problem by giving prevalence figures for osteoporosis, data on hospital admissions related to osteoporosis, and figures on the cost to the nation of the problem.

Don't baffle your readers

Although you don't want to patronise and bore your readers by telling them things that they already know, you certainly don't want to baffle them by introducing, without explanation, material that is wholly unfamiliar. Nothing turns readers off faster than abbreviations that mean nothing or references to diseases, drugs, reports, places, or whatever that they do not know. This point simply emphasises the importance of knowing your audience.

Give the study's design but not the conclusion

This is a matter of choice, but I asked authors to give a one sentence description of their study at the end of the introduction. The last line might read:

> We therefore conducted a double blind randomised study with
> 10-year follow up to determine whether teetotallers drinking
> three glasses of whisky a week can reduce their chances of dying
> of coronary artery disease.

I don't like it, however, when the introduction also gives the final conclusion:

> Drinking three glasses of whisky a week does not reduce teetotallers'
> chances of dying of coronary artery disease.

Other editors may think differently.

Think about using journalistic tricks sparingly

The difficult part of writing is to get the structure right. Spinning sentences is much easier than finding the right structure, and editors can much more easily change sentences than structure. Most pieces of writing that fail do so because the structure is poor and that is why writing scientific articles is comparatively easy – the structure is given to you.

I have assumed in this chapter that you are writing a scientific paper. If you are writing something else you will have to think much harder about the introduction and about the structure of the whole piece. But even if you are writing a scientific paper you might make use of the devices that journalists use to hook their readers.

Tim Albert, a medical journalist, gives five possible openings in his excellent book on medical journalism [15]: telling an arresting story, describing a scene vividly, using a strong quotation, giving some intriguing facts, or making an opinionated and controversial pronouncement. He gives two examples from the health page of *The Independent*. Mike Hanscomb wrote:

> In many respects it is easier and less uncomfortable to have leukaemia than eczema?

This is an intriguing statement and readers will be interested to read on to see if the author can convince them that his statement contains some truth. Jeremy Laurance began a piece:

> This is a story of sex, fear, and money. It is about a new treatment for an embarrassing problem which could prove a money spinner in the new commercial National Health Service?

Sex, fear, and money are emotive to all of us and we may well want to know how a new treatment could make money for the health service rather than costing it money. My favourite beginning occurs in Anthony Burgess's novel *Earthly Powers*. The first sentence reads:

> It was the afternoon of my eighty-first birthday, and I was in bed with my catamite when Ali announced that the archbishop had come to see me.

This starts the book so powerfully that it might well carry us right through the next 400 or so pages. (I had to look up 'catamite' too. It means 'boy kept for homosexual purposes'.)

To begin a paper in the *British Journal of Anaesthesia* with such a sentence would be to court rejection, ridicule, and disaster, but some of the techniques advocated by Tim Albert could be used. I suggest, however, staying away from opinionated statements and quotations in scientific papers, particularly if they come from Shakespeare, the Bible, or *Alice in Wonderland*.

Conclusion

To write an effective introduction you must know your audience, keep it short, tell readers why you have done the study and explain why it's important, convince them that it is better than what has gone before, and try as hard as you can to hook them in the first line.

References

1 Chalmers I. Improving the quality and dissemination of reviews of clinical research. In: Lock S, ed., *The future of medical journals*. London: BMJ Books, 1991, pp. 127–48.

2 Mulrow CD. The medical review article: state of the science. *Ann Intern Med* 1987; **104**:485–8.

3 World Medical Association. Declaration of Helsinki. Recommendations guiding physicians in biomedical research involving human subjects. *JAMA* 1997; **277**:925–6.

4 Moher D, Schulz KF, Altman DG. The CONSORT statement: revised recommendations for improving the quality of reports of parallel-group randomised trials. *Lancet* 2001;**357**:1191–4.

5 Lau J, Antman EM, Jimenez-Silva J, Kupelnick B, Mosteller F, Chalmers TC. Cumulative meta-analysis of therapeutic trials for myocardial infarction. *New Engl J Med* 1992;**327**:248–54.

6 Bero L, Delamothe T, Dixon A, *et al.* The electronic future: what might an online scientific paper look like in five years' time? *BMJ* 1997;**315**:1692–6.

7 Delamothe T. Is that it? How online articles have changed over the past five years. *BMJ* 2002;**325**:1475–8.

8 Müllner M, Groves T. Making research papers in the BMJ more accessible. *BMJ* 2002;**325**:456.

9 Smith R. Scientific articles have hardly changed in 50 years. *BMJ* 2004;**328**:1533.

10 Doll R, Peto R, Boreham J, Sutherland I. Mortality in relation to smoking: 50 years' observations on male British doctors. *BMJ* 2004;**328**:1519–33.

11 Doll R, Hill AB. The mortality of doctors in relation to their smoking habits. A preliminary report. *BMJ* 1954;**228**(i):1451–5.

12 Moher D, Cook DJ, Eastwood S, Olkin I, Rennie D, Stroup DF. Improving the quality of reports of meta-analyses of randomised controlled trials: the QUOROMstatement. Quality of reporting of meta-analyses. *Lancet* 1999;**354**:1896–900.

13 Drummond MF, Jefferson TO. Guidelines for authors and peer reviewers of economic submissions to the BMJ. The BMJ economic evaluation working party. *BMJ* 1996;**313**:275–83.

14 Bossuyt PM, Reitsma B, Brns DE, *et al.* Towards complete and accurate reporting of studies of diagnostic accuracy: the STARD initiative. *BMJ* 2003;**326**:41–4.

15 Albert T. *Medical journalism: the writer's guide*. Oxford: Radcliffe, 1992.

Chapter 3 **Methods**

Gordon B. Drummond

You should describe, in logical sequence, how your study was designed and carried out, and how you analysed your data. If the study is already finished, this should be a simple task. However, do not leave writing the methods until this stage! The sooner you write down the methods, the sooner you can detect and deal with flaws in the design. Write it down, in full detail, *before you start the study* and ask an experienced colleague to look it over. The challenge of setting down what you intend to do is also a very useful exercise – far better than discovering predictable flaws after months of hard work. In fact, if you are conducting a therapeutic trial, you will have to register the study, and its methods, before you start. If you don't, many journals will not publish it.

Testing hypotheses

When readers turn to the methods section, they look for more than details of the apparatus or assay that you used. The methods section should answer the questions 'Who, what, why, when, and where?' Even more important, it should state the hypothesis that was tested – for example, that a treatment has a particular effect, such as increased survival or improved outcome. This is formally tested by assuming that the null hypothesis is true. The observed results indicate how tenable this hypothesis can be – that is, the possibility that the intervention was without effect. Naturally, we would hope that this possibility would be small (much less than 1, which is complete certainty). We state how small this possibility (p-value) has to be to disprove the null hypothesis as the 'mission statement' of the study. A study of two antibiotics might compare cure rates. The null hypothesis is that there is no difference between these rates. The statistical tests used will estimate the likelihood that the rates are statistically indistinguishable (the rates one might expect if the drugs had been the same, so that both samples were treated equally). A p-value of less than 0.05 (out of a total probability of 1) shows that the possibility that the rates were statistically similar would have been found in less than 1 out of 20 experiments. Many papers merely say, adequately, '$p<0.05$ was considered significant'.

The other side of the coin of probability, often neglected, is the *power* of the study. If the null hypothesis survives attempts to destroy its credibility, you cannot conclude immediately that there is no difference between the groups. You have only concluded that the rates are statistically indistinguishable. Are your methods sufficiently exacting to test the null hypothesis properly? A true difference might indeed be present, but it could be small. Another possibility is that a difference may exist, but because the measurements vary, the variations swamp the effect you seek. In both cases, a small 'signal-to-noise' ratio is present. You must therefore also estimate the power of the study to detect what you are looking for, to indicate possibility of a false negative result. This is the β error. The value you choose depends on factors such as the precision of the answer needed and may also take into account the practical consequences of an incorrect conclusion. A β-value is often taken as 0.2, which implies a *power* of 0.8 to avoid a false negative result. In practice, the power of a study depends on the size of the effect, the variability of the data, and the number of observations. A power of 0.8 is often taken as adequate, but this may not always be sensible: take advice if you are unhappy with a false negative result.

Always state clearly the *a priori* hypotheses – if only to be sure that you collect appropriate and relevant data and do the correct statistical tests.

Statistics

State the exact tests used to analyse the data, and include an appropriate reference if the test is not well known. State the software, and the version, that you used. The statistical test you should use depends on the type of data. Sometimes the distribution of the data may not be clear before the study is over, so the *a priori* tests should be chosen conservatively and be non-parametric.

Design

The study design can often be described with a few well-chosen words, particularly if it is a description of the layout of groups or events. The groups may be *independent*, allocated to different treatments, and the design is often *parallel*, where each group receives a different treatment and all groups enter at the same time. In this case, comparisons will be between groups. Participants who receive different treatments may be paired to reduce the effects of confounding variables, such as weight or sex. The effects of a treatment on each participant may be assessed before and after; such comparisons are *within subject*. The simplest study design is a *randomised parallel design*, with a comparison of outcome between groups (Box 3.1).

Box 3.1 What to include in the methods section

How the study was designed
- Keep the description brief
- Say how randomisation was done
- Use names to identify parts of a study sequence

How the study was carried out
- Describe how the participants were recruited and chosen
- Give reasons for excluding participants
- Consider mentioning ethical features
- Give accurate details of materials used
- Give exact drug dosages
- Give the exact form of treatment and accessible details of unusual apparatus

How the data were analysed
- Use a *p*-value to disprove the null hypothesis
- Give an estimate of the power of the study (the likelihood of a false negative – the β error)
- Give the exact tests used for statistical analysis (chosen *a priori*)

Always state clearly how randomisation was done, because this is a crucial part of many clinical trials. The method used should be stated explicitly. Describe any specific aspects such as blocked randomisation (to obtain roughly similar group sizes) and stratification (to obtain a balance of confounding variables, such as age or sex, in each group). Authors often get randomisation wrong, by using alternate cases, unit number, date of birth, and so on. Correct methods involve the use of random number tables or closed envelopes. If assessment of the outcome is blinded, try to describe how the assessor was kept unaware of the treatment allocation. If blinding is important, you should be able to show that all who took part remained unaware of the allocation. To do this, ask them to guess the allocation after the study is over, and then test to see if the guess rate is better than that expected by chance alone.

A diagram can help a lot to describe a complex study design or sequence of interventions. Help your readers to follow the results by using explicit names for separate groups or parts of a study sequence. Initials, or even short names, are a clearer way to designate such groups or events than calling them 1, 2, and 3.

Participants and materials

Readers should know how the participants were recruited and chosen. A study of healthy, non-pregnant (probably male) volunteers may not indicate the effects of the drug on old ladies. State if subjects with specific diseases have been excluded and how these diseases were defined and diagnosed. Were subjects already on medication excluded from the study? Alcohol and tobacco use can alter drug responses, and it is tempting to exclude participants who drink and smoke, but the results in such cases would be less applicable to clinical practice. Listing the inclusion and exclusion criteria set out in the ethics application form is important.

Although most journals indicate that ethical approval is a prerequisite for acceptance, some ethical features of the study design may need to be mentioned. For example, you may need to describe some of the practical problems of obtaining informed consent or a satisfactory comparative treatment. Keep a note of eligible participants who are approached and then decide not to take part: are there many of these, and are they different from the participants who agree to take part?

In a laboratory study, you must detail the source and strain of animals, bacteria, or other biological material, or the raw materials used. Such information is necessary to allow comparisons with other studies and to allow others to repeat the study you have described. Give exact drug dosages (generic name, chemical formula if not well known, and the proprietary preparation used) and how you prepared solutions, with their precise concentrations.

The exact form of treatment used has to be described in a way that allows replication. If the methods, devices, or techniques are widely known or can be looked up in a standard text – for example, the random zero sphygmomanometer or a Vitalograph spirometer – further information is unnecessary. Similarly, a widely used apparatus, such as the Fleisch pneumotachograph, does not require further description, but less well-known apparatus should be described by giving the name, type, and manufacturer.

Describe fully any methods that are uncommon or unique, or provide an adequate accessible reference to the method. Readers will justifiably object if a reference is only to an abstract or a limited description in a previous paper. If in doubt, provide details and indicate how the methods were validated.

Describe the apparatus used in sufficient detail to allow the reader to be confident of the results reported. Is the apparatus appropriate, sensitive enough, specific in its measurement, reproducible, and accurate? Each aspect may need to be considered separately. For example, bathroom scales may fulfil all of these criteria when used to estimate human body weight, as long as they have been checked and calibrated recently. On the other hand, an inadequate chemical assay may be non-specific because it responds to other substances, gives different results when the same sample is tested twice (poor reproducibility), or gives results that consistently are different from the value expected when tested with a standard substance (poor accuracy). The method may not detect low concentrations (insufficient sensitivity). Any of these faults could invalidate a study.

You may need to describe how you calibrated, standardised, and checked the linearity and frequency response of the measuring devices used. Do not merely repeat the manufacturer's data for accuracy of a piece of apparatus, particularly if it is crucial to the study: the standard used for calibration must be stated and the results of the calibration quoted. If analogue to digital conversion is done for computer analysis, the sampling rate and the accuracy of the sampling must be given.

Adequate descriptions are needed for all methods of assessment and follow up. Methods such as questionnaires should have been validated, and data collection and transcription should be checked (Box 3.2).

Box 3.2 A good methods section can answer these questions

- Does the text describe what question was being asked, what was being tested, and how trustworthy the measurements are?
- Were the measurements recorded, analysed, and interpreted correctly?
- Would a suitably qualified reader be able to repeat the experiment in the same way?

Recommended reading

DeAngelis CD, Drazen JM, Frizelle FA, *et al.* Clinical trial registration – a statement from the International Committee of Medical Journal Editors. *JAMA-J Am Med Assoc* 2004;**292**:1363–4.

Eger EI. A template for writing a scientific paper. *Anesth Analog* 1990;**70**:91–6.

Grimes DA, Schulz KF. Descriptive studies: what they can and cannot do. *Lancet* 2002;**359**:14.

Moher D, Schulz KF, Altman DG, for the CONSORT group. The CONSORT statement: revised recommendations for improving the quality of reports of parallel-group randomised trials. *Lancet* 2001;**357**:1191–4.

Chapter 4 **Results**

Hans-Joachim Priebe

The results section answers the question 'What was found?' It reports the results of the investigation(s) described in the methods section, and it usually does not contain interpretation of data or statements that require referencing. It is composed of words (they tell the story), tables (that summarise the evidence), illustrations (that highlight the main findings), and statistics (that support the statements).

Pay special attention to two pieces of general advice. Firstly, *keep the results section as brief and uncluttered as possible.* The reader must be able to see the wood for the trees. Report only the results that are relevant to the question and hypothesis posed in the introduction section. Secondly, *organise the presentation of results.* Design the text as if you were telling the reader a story. Start chronologically and continue logically to the end. Lead the reader through the story by using a mixture of text, tables, and illustrations.

The words

Start the results section by characterising the participants and objects of your study in enough detail for the reader to assess how representative they were and, if more than one group was studied, how comparable they were. You need to confirm that the participants were comparable, even if they were assigned randomly to the groups. If the groups differ in any way, you will have to comment in the discussion section on how the differences might have affected your results. Items under investigation – for example, bacterial species investigated or substance used – should be mentioned at least once, preferably in the first sentence. When you identify individual participants, use A, B, C, etc. or 1, 2, 3, etc. (when more than 26 subjects) rather than the participant's initials. Do not call the characteristics of subjects the 'demographics'.

Continue the section by presenting the answers to your main questions. Report results that do not support or that even refute your original hypothesis. Such unexpected results may generate new ideas and can avoid unnecessary future studies. Avoid the much dreaded (by editor, assessor, and reader) statement: 'The results are presented in tables X–Z and in figures A–C'. Such a statement does not contain any relevant information. On the contrary, it leaves the reader searching for the meaningful result.

Address one topic per paragraph – from most important to least important. Preferably, place those results that directly answer the question posed at the beginning of the results section and of successive paragraphs. Start the paragraph with a topic sentence – a sentence that states the topic or message of the paragraph. The topic is what the paragraph is about, and the message is the point the paragraph is making.

Differentiate clearly between results and data. Results are not identical with data. *Data* are factual findings (often numbers) derived from measurements and observations. Data can be raw (e.g. all blood pressure measurements during an investigation), summarised (e.g. mean and standard deviation), or transformed (e.g. percentage of baseline condition). *Results*, in contrast, state the meaning of the data (e.g. 'Furosemide administered during mechanical ventilation increased urine output').

Data can rarely be listed without stating the result. For example, consider the following statement: 'In 14 untreated individuals, the mean blood glucose concentration was 205 ± 10 (SD) mg%. In 16 patients treated with drug X, the mean blood glucose concentration was 105 ± 10 mg%'. The implication of the data is not immediately obvious. The reader is forced to draw their own conclusion, which makes it more difficult for them to read and understand.

Consider a revised version of the same results. 'The mean blood glucose concentration was 50% lower in the 16 patients treated with drug X than in the 14 untreated individuals (105 ± 10 (SD) versus 205 ± 10 mg%, $p < 0.001$)'. This sentence states both the data and the results. The reader now receives immediate information on the direction ('was lower'), the magnitude ('50%'), and the likelihood of a chance finding ('$p < 0.001$') of the observed difference.

Emphasise important results by omitting data from the text, condensing the results, using a result as a topic sentence, putting the most important results at the beginning of a paragraph, and subordinating less important information. Remember that having to sort through a lot of data in the text makes for difficult reading, so data (especially when numerous) are often presented in tables and figures. Avoid duplicating data that are depicted in tables and figures in the text. If several variables change in the same direction, report the resulting change for all variables once rather than the same change variable by variable.

Do not use table headings or figure legends as topic sentences. State the results directly and cite (in parentheses) figures and tables after the first mention of results relevant to the figure or table. For example, consider the following statement: 'Systemic haemodynamic data are summarised in Figure 3. Inhalational agent X (1.5 MAC) decreased cardiac output, systemic blood pressure, systemic vascular resistance, and heart rate'. The first sentence repeats a figure legend ('Figure 3, Systemic haemodynamic data') and merely indicates the topic – systemic haemodynamic data. After reading the first sentence, the reader has no idea what message to expect in the figure. Only the second sentence carries a message in which the reader is interested – systemic haemodynamic variables decreased. Furthermore, an entire sentence is wasted just on pointing the reader towards a figure.

Consider the revision: 'Inhalational agent X (1.5 MAC) decreased cardiac output, systemic blood pressure, systemic vascular resistance, and heart rate (Figure 3)'. After reading this sentence, the reader has a clear expectation when turning to the stated figure – decreases in all haemodynamic variables.

Report the results of discrete events in the *past tense*, because they occurred in the past (e.g. 'Inhalational agent X inhibited hypoxic pulmonary vasoconstriction'). Report results of a descriptive nature in the *present tense*, because the described state continues to be true. When comparing results, use 'than' not 'compared with'. For example, the statement 'X was decreased compared with Y' is ambiguous. It can mean 'X was lower than Y', 'X decreased more than Y', or 'X decreased but Y remained unchanged'. State unambiguously what you mean to say.

Be precise in your choice of words. The implication of 'We were unable to identify the existence of substance X in material Y' is clearly different from 'No substance X was found in material Y'. The first statement addresses the issue of ability and implies that substance X may actually exist in material Y but, for whatever reason (like inadequate sensitivity of method), you were not able to identify it. The second statement addresses the issue of actuality and implies that no substance X is present in material Y and thus would not be detected whatever technique was used. Choose the verb according to whether you want to address ability or actuality.

Similarly, the implication of the statement 'Substance X *did not* decrease systemic vascular resistance' is clearly different from that of 'Substance X *failed* to decrease systemic vascular resistance'. 'Failed' implies that you actually had expected a decrease in systemic vascular resistance. 'Did not' implies no such *a priori* expectation. 'Did not decrease' is the usual preferred form used to describe results.

Avoid the use of qualitative words such as 'markedly' and 'significantly'. The reader cannot judge the actual magnitude of a 'marked' decrease in systemic blood pressure. Unless accompanied by quantitative data (such as percentage changes) in text, tables or figures, qualitative descriptions are subject to individual judgement. Furthermore, the word 'significant' has become a synonym for 'statistically significant' and thus can no longer be used interchangeably with 'markedly'. The wording 'Systemic blood pressure decreased significantly' asks for statistical data to support such a statement.

Tables and illustrations: general considerations

Keep in mind that many readers tend to skip the text or read only part of it. They prefer looking at tables and illustrations, it is important therefore that tables and illustrations have strong visual impact, are informative and easy to comprehend, and can stand alone. Readers must be able to interpret them without needing to refer to the text or to other figures and tables. This requires careful design, informative legends for figures, and informative titles and footnotes for tables.

Tables and illustrations should follow a sequence that clearly relates to the text and tells the story of the paper. Design figures and tables and figure legends and footnotes in parallel, so as to prepare the reader for the next table or illustration. Use identical names of variables, units of measurements, and abbreviations in text, tables, and illustrations.

Use the fewest tables and illustrations needed to tell the story. Do not duplicate data in tables and illustrations. It is acceptable to summarise data in tables or illustrations, and to present primary evidence (e.g. a single recording of an electroencephalogram) in a separate figure.

Strictly follow the journal's 'Instructions to authors'. Should you have the misfortune to have your paper refused by one journal, check the instructions and modify the paper before submitting to a second journal. Remember editors and assessors may not look kindly on material that is obviously in the format of another journal.

The tables

In the results section, tables present data that support results. In this context, they serve two main purposes: to present individual data for all subjects and objects studied or to make a point by presenting summary data (e.g. means with standard deviations). Each table should deal with a specific problem.

All tables are basically structured the same way, with four main parts: title, column headings, body, and footnotes. Keep the title brief, and ensure that it relates clearly to the content of the table. Use identical key terms in the title and column headings, or use a category term (e.g. 'Effects of inhalational anaesthetic X on systemic haemodynamics') in the title rather than repeating several column headings (e.g. 'Effects of inhalational anaesthetic

X on arterial blood pressure, central venous pressure, cardiac output, and systemic vascular resistance').

The *column headings* consist of headings that identify the items listed in the columns below, subheadings (if required), and units of measurement (if required). Keep column headings brief. For experiments that have independent and dependent variables, the independent variable is in the left column, and the dependent variable in the right column. The sample size (n) can form an additional type of column heading and column.

A table with many dependent variables would become too wide for a page if dependent variables were listed across the top. Placing standard deviations, standard errors of the mean, confidence intervals, or ranges below the mean may solve this problem in some but not all cases. In this instance, consider switching the position of independent and dependent variables. The dependent variables then would be listed down the first column on the left, and the independent variables across the top.

Use *subheadings* to subdivide a heading into further categories. List (mostly in parentheses) the units of measurement after or below the name of the variable in the column heading. Do not repeat them after each value. Use the International System of Units (SI) abbreviations for units of measurement. Make an effort to use units of measurement that avoid listing numerous zeros (e.g. '28 km' rather than '28 000 m'). However, avoid the use of multipliers in column headings (e.g. '$\times 10^{4}$') as a means of eliminating zeros. Multipliers are confusing: is the reader supposed to multiply by 10^{4} or has the author already done so?

The *body of the table* consists of columns (vertically listed items and data) and rows (horizontally listed items and data). The column on the left lists the items (usually the independent variables) for which data are listed, and the columns on the right list the corresponding data.

Placement of standard deviations can be difficult, especially in the case of several columns. If placed to the right of the mean, reading and comparison of standard deviations across rows are hindered. Likewise, if the standard deviations are placed below the mean, reading and comparison along rows are hindered. If you prefer the reader to make crosswise comparisons, then place the standard deviations below the mean. If you think that lengthwise comparisons are more informative, then place the standard deviations next to the mean. Placing the standard deviations below the mean has the advantage of reducing the width of the table. If you remain unsatisfied with either solution, consider putting the standard deviations in parentheses instead of using $\pm$.

Use the fewest decimal places needed to convey the precision of the measurement. Use the same number of decimal places in means and standard deviations. In each column, align the data on the decimal point (irrespective of whether or not a decimal point is present) and on the ± (e.g. when data are presented as mean ± standard deviations).

Tables are a visual medium, so indicate statistically significant differences between data by placing symbols (e.g. asterisks (*)) after values that are different, and then define the symbols in the footnote. Do not place symbols after control values or between two values. Adding a separate column of p-values is not advantageous, because symbols have a greater visual impact and add less bulk to the body of the table. You do not need to identify nonsignificant differences. As much as a * in a column of aligned numbers is a clear signal of a statistically significant difference, so the absence of a * is a clear signal for the lack of such difference. In addition, NS (for 'not significant') is not informative, because the p-value could have been 0.06 or 0.9.

Usually, a table should include enough data to make it more efficient than listing the numbers in the text. At the same time, it should be small and concise enough to be easily readable. If you have only a small amount of data, list the values in the text. If a table is too large, delete unnecessary columns (e.g. a column of p-values) and rows; avoid repetition of information; keep titles, headings, and subheadings brief; use abbreviations (and explain them in the footnotes); and consider splitting one excessively large table into two smaller tables.

Although certain aspects of table format differ between journals, some generally accepted standards exist. Three horizontal lines are usually used to separate parts of the table: one above the column headings, one below the column headings, and one below the data (to separate the body of the table from the footnotes). In tables with subheadings, short horizontal lines are used to group the subheadings under the respective heading. Avoid (unless requested by a journal's instructions to authors) the use of additional horizontal (between row) and vertical (between column) lines because they give the table a cluttered appearance.

If you want the reader to look at changes, remember that most readers in the Western World read naturally from left to right, not from top to bottom. The results should thus be presented in columns in which the changes run from the left-most column. Often, it helps to present results as percentage changes from the initial value. If you do this, include an initial column of actual data as well.

Tables 4.1 and 4.2 illustrate what is often submitted and how the information can be made to look much better.

Table 4.1 is an example of a poor table. The title does not explain the initiating stimulus to the observed responses. It lists individual haemodynamic variables rather than using a category term. The 'condition' is poorly

Table 4.1 Heart rate, blood pressure, and cardiac output responses

Condition	Heart rate	Systolic BP	Diastolic BP	Cardiac output
Awake	71 ± 10	130 ± 12	84 ± 9	4264 ± 0692
Anaesthesia	69 ± 7	112 ± 10	69 ± 8	3575 ± 0588
Sternotomy	93 ± 12	177 ± 17	106 ± 13	4471 ± 0.934
Anaesthesia	79 ± 9	127 ± 12	76 ± 10	3986 ± 0765

BP: blood pressure.

defined. All of the vertical and most of the horizontal grid lines are superfluous. The columns have no indication of the units used. The results for cardiac output show more decimal places than the precision of the measurement justifies. The ± value is not defined (is it standard deviation or standard error of the mean?). No mention is made of the number of participants studied. The changes run from top to bottom rather than from left to right across the page. Abbreviations are not explained. No indication is given of any statistically significant changes.

Consider now a revised version of the same table (Table 4.2). When considered in combination with the footnote, this table provides all the information needed by the reader. The title describes the initiating stimuli ('Induction of anaesthesia and sternotomy') and uses a category term ('cardiovascular'). The superfluous grid lines are eliminated. Changes run across the table from

Table 4.2 Cardiovascular responses to induction of anaesthesia and sternotomy

	Induction of anaesthesia		Sternotomy	
	Before	After	During	After
Heart rate	71 ± 10	69 ± 7	93 ± 12*	79 ± 9
(beats/min)	(59–100)	(53–89)	(69–130)	(61–101)
Systolic BP	130 ± 12	112 ± 10*	177 ± 17*	127 + 12
(mmHg)	(101–148)	(85–139)	(121–209)	(94–149)
Diastolic BP	84 ± 9	69 ± 8*	106 ± 13*	76 ± 10
(mmHg)	(64–103)	(50–89)	(83–131)	(58–100)
Cardiac output	4.3 ± 0.7	3.6 ± 0.6*	4.5 + 0.9	4.0 ± 0.8
(l/min)	(3.1–5.9)	(2.6–4.9)	(3.0–6.1)	(2.9–5.2)

BP: blood pressure.
Data are means ± SD (range) obtained in 11 patients 5 min before and after induction of anaesthesia, and during and 5 min after sternotomy.
*$p < 0.05$ versus 'before induction of anaesthesia' by ANOVA.

the left-most column. The subheadings ('Before', 'After', 'During', and 'After') allow clear chronological allocation of observation points. Units of measurement are provided. The asterisks in two columns are a clear signal of a statistically significant difference (the absence is a clear signal for the lack of such a difference). The footnote defines the kind of data, the number of patients studied, the observation points, the abbreviations, the statistical significance level, and the statistics used. This table can now stand on its own. Your reader will be able to obtain all the information they need without having to refer back to the text.

The illustrations

The main purpose of illustrations in the results section is to present evidence that supports the results – either as primary evidence (e.g. electrocardiographs or radiographs) or as numerical data (e.g. graphs or histograms).

Ensure good readability. Remember that illustrations have to go through a number of processes before appearing in print. With each process, some detail will be lost, so make sure the quality of your originals is as good as possible. Check legibility by reducing the figure to publication size with a photocopier. The smallest letter should be at least 1.5 mm high. Symbols must be large enough to be identified easily. Emphasise important information by using different line weights. Make each figure deliver a clear message. Only some key points can be given here, so use Tufte's books (see the recommended reading list), which are excellent guides as to what can and should be done.

Present primary evidence when this is the type of data you have or when you want to show the quality of your data acquisition. For example, a paper reporting an investigation on coronary blood flow, in addition to summarising your data in numerical form (e.g. in graphs or tables), could show a representative coronary blood flow recording. Select the best quality recording for reproduction.

Label your illustrations adequately. The extent of labelling depends on the readership. The more general the readership, the more labelling usually is required. Labels include arrows, arrowheads, letters, numbers, and symbols. Define the labels in the figure legend. Use the fewest, briefest, and smallest labels possible.

Figure legends

A figure legend is a descriptive statement that is placed next to the figure. It is essential to make the figure understandable without the reader needing to refer to the text. The type of figure will determine the content of the figure legend, which typically consists of up to four parts: a brief title, experimental details, various definitions (e.g. of symbols or abbreviations), and statistical information.

Keep the title brief, use the same key terms that you use in the figures and text, and avoid the use of abbreviations. Where appropriate, provide just enough experimental detail to allow the reader to understand the figure. Define symbols or line patterns by redrawing them in the figure legend. Make sure that the patterns in the legend match the patterns in illustrations. If identical symbols or abbreviations are used in several figures, define them the first time they occur and then refer the reader to the legend that contains the definitions.

The statistical information required in the figure legend depends on the type of illustration. Information for graphs should include whether data represent individual, mean, or median values; whether error bars represent standard deviations (SD), standard errors of the mean (SEM), confidence intervals (CI), or ranges; and the sample size (n). For bar graphs, state which values were compared by statistical analysis, the significance value (p-value), and possibly the statistical test you used. Avoid writing '$n =11$', as such statements may be ambiguous; be more specific – for example, write '11 blood samples', '11 measurements', or '11 rats'. In addition to this standard structure of a figure legend, the legend can point to an unusual or interesting finding.

When you use photographs of patients, you must obtain written, informed consent before an individual's photograph is taken and published. Cover facial features whenever possible. Use A, B, etc., not initials, when you need to refer to a patient.

When using polygraph recordings, eliminate grid lines, and add vertical and horizontal scales. Make sure that scales and scale markers are absolutely accurate. Label each scale marker with the appropriate unit. Use the SI abbreviations for units of measurement.

Many types of graphs are available, so carefully choose the graph that best represents your data. In line graphs, the independent variable (e.g. time) is conventionally on the x-axis and the dependent variable (e.g. blood pressure) on the y-axis. If the scale is linear, tick marks and scale numbers must be spaced at equal distances and intervals, respectively, starting where the axes meet. In a bar graph, the axis must include zero, otherwise, the differences between bars are obscured. As the baseline is not an axis, so no line or tick marks are needed along the baseline.

Republishing figures

You need to first obtain permission from the copyright holder (usually the publisher) – this is a legal requirement. You should also obtain permission from the author, as common courtesy. Standard permission forms are available from publishers.

Give attribution to the source and the publisher. Cite the reference in the figure legend and state that you have permission for republication. Credit is always given at the very end of a figure legend. Attribution can read as follows: 'From Laver *et al.* (1981), with permission', or 'From Ref. [10], with permission from the *British Journal of Anaesthesia*'. When you have modified an original illustration, the attribution could read: 'Redrawn from Laver *et al.* (1981); reproduced with permission'.

The statistics

Statistics must accompany data. Many papers suffer because the statistics are badly presented. Obviously, many statistical tests exist – conventional as well as esoteric. Choose the test most appropriate for your data analysis. Decide on which statistical test to use when planning your study. Do not take the data of your finished study to your local statistician to see what can be made of them – that is a waste of everyone's time.

Follow some general rules. As data are mostly restricted to tables and figures, that is where you should include most statistical data. Specify the type of statistic, the sample size (n), and the probability value for a test of statistical significance (p-value). When normally distributed data have been analysed statistically, report the mean and a statistic that indicates the variation from the mean (e.g. the standard deviation or the range). When non-normally distributed data have been analysed statistically, report the median and the interquartile range (the range between the 25th and the 75th percentiles).

When you list statistical details in the text, follow some conventional rules. Mean and standard deviation are usually written as '11.4 $\pm$ 0.8 (SD) kg'. The conventional way to write data that are being compared statistically is: 'Body weight increased more in group A than in group B (13.2 $\pm$ 1.9 (SD) versus 9.4 $\pm$ 0.9 kg in eight patients, $p < 0.02$)'. This statement contains five types of statistical information: the mean ('13.2' and '9.4 kg'), the standard deviation ('1.9' and '0.9'), specification of the statistic used to describe the variation from the mean ('SD'), the sample size (n) ('8 patients'), and the probability value of significance ('$p < 0.02$'). Usually, you should provide all five types of statistical information; however, if any of these statistical parameters apply to all data (e.g. SD and sample size), you only need to describe the complete statistical details when you list the data the first time and can omit thereafter those that apply to all data. If you decide to report the confidence interval, the statement can be rewritten as follows: 'Body weight increased more in group A than in group B (13.2 $\pm$ 1.9 (SD) versus 9.4 $\pm$ 0.9 kg in eight patients; 95% confidence interval for the difference = 1.8 – 5.2 kg, $p < 0.02$)'.

When you provide p-values, you should list the actual p-values not only for those differences considered statistically significant (e.g. $p < 0.02$), but also for differences not considered significant (e.g. $p > 0.6$ or $p = 0.55$). By restricting the information to statements like '$p > 0.05$' or '$p =$ NS', you restrict the reader's ability to interpret the data accurately: a p-value of 0.06 does not exclude the possibility of a statistically significant difference as strongly as a p-value of >0.9.

Do not list data to a greater degree of accuracy than that of the measurement. For example, if you can measure cardiac output with an accuracy of only $\pm10\%$, do not quote values for individual results to three decimal places. Make sure that any change described as statistically significant is greater than the error of your measurement. Be particularly careful with calculated values: the errors of the original measurements add up alarmingly.

Take care when you look at associations between variables. Statistical significance needs to indicate how much of an association can be attributed to the dependency of one variable on another and how much is due to chance. Be careful with extrapolation, and do not confuse association with causation.

Statistical presentation is always a problem – too much information, too little space. Present enough information for the intelligent reader to believe what you are saying. Remember: usually, neither your readers, nor your assessors, are expert statisticians. If your statistical tests are too esoteric, be prepared for a lengthy discussion before publication.

Conclusion

The results section is the easiest to write. The introduction has defined the questions and the methods the means of getting the answers. Decide during the design stage of your study how the results will be presented. Apart from filling in the actual data in the tables and placing the actual dots and lines in the figures, you could almost write the results as you start the investigation. Remember to follow the general design of the results section: the text should tell the story, the tables will summarise the evidence, the illustrations will show the highlights, and the statistics should support your statements. Keep it all straightforward – and always keep the reader in mind.

Recommended reading

Huth EJ. *Writing and publishing in medicine*. Baltimore: Williams & Wilkens, 1999. (An excellent book about the process of writing and publishing.)

O'Connor M. *Writing successfully in science*. London: Chapman & Hall, 1991. (An excellent guide to the topic.)

Tufte ER. *The visual display of quantitative information.* Cheshire, CT: Graphics Press, 1983. (This book shows what is too often done and what can be done.)

Tufte ER. *Visual explanations.* Cheshire, CT: Graphics Press, 1997. (This is a guide on how to use graphics and to get your point across.)

Zeiger M. *Essentials of writing biomedical research papers.* New York: McGrawHill, 2000. (An outstanding guide to good scientific writing that contains numerous exercises.)

Chapter 5 **Discussion**

George M. Hall

Many authors find this section of the paper to be the most difficult. However, it should be an exercise in logic and discipline and a satisfactory discussion can be based on the format shown in Box 5.1. Poor discussions have no structure, try to cite all publications found during the literature search and induce acute boredom in the reader. Keep it short, snappy and relevant. A useful rule is – if in doubt cut it out. You are most unlikely to have a manuscript rejected just because the discussion is too short.

Box 5.1 Discussion: overall format

- Statement of principal finding(s)
- Appraisal of methods
- Comparison with previous work
- Clinical and scientific implications (if any)
- Further work
- ? Conclusion
- Acknowledgements

Principal findings

The reader has just finished a detailed presentation of the results so it is important to remind them of the key findings. A good start to the discussion is two or three sentences that summarise the results. These should be clear and unambiguous, the 'take home message', and can often be used in the abstract. Further analysis of the data should not be undertaken in the discussion. If you missed something important out of the results then you will have to go back and rewrite this section.

Methodology

It is most unlikely that the methods used in the study were perfect so a brief appraisal is necessary in the discussion. A common problem is the sample size and the power calculation described in the methods may have been optimistic. There is no point in trying to hide this from editors and assessors. It may be necessary to down grade your study from the definitive clinical trial in this area to a pilot or preliminary study that will enable other researchers to undertake a correctly powered investigation.

Unusual study designs often alarm assessors so you should explain precisely why you chose this design and, if possible, provide supporting citations using similar methodology. To use a sporting analogy, 'get your retaliation in first'. In essence, you are trying to deal with any criticisms from editors and assessors by showing that you had already thought of the difficulties inherent in the study design.

On the other hand you may be able to emphasise here any strengths of the methods used. For example, you may have developed a more sensitive and specific assay for plasma rhubarb concentrations that has enabled you to find changes during routine surgery that other investigators failed to observe. Criticism of the methodology of previous investigators may be appropriate, but make sure that you remain objective and scrupulously fair.

Previous work

A key part of the discussion is the comparison of your results with other published studies. You should cite only major relevant work, both confirmatory and contradictory. Do not simply repeat the sentences you used in the introduction when defining the research question, and never, never quote what you have not read. There is the temptation to cite every paper written on the subject to show the assessors the thoroughness of your literature search. Resist the temptation, a surfeit of references is a sign of insecurity not scholarship. You will know who are the major research groups so concentrate on them. Do not ignore previous literature that disagrees with your findings. This 'selective citation' will be spotted very quickly by assessors and you will lose credibility as a consequence. When dealing with previous work be impartial, there are often good reasons why results cannot be exactly replicated and you may be able to explain some of the discrepancies.

Implications

If your results may change clinical practice, then this should be discussed. Most investigators never make a major breakthrough so do not exaggerate the importance of your work. It is likely to be just a small contribution to a limited area of knowledge, but it is still important to state how our understanding has increased as a result of your work. If there has been no progress, it indicates that the study was of little value. Similarly, if the study was non-clinical, any basic scientific implications should be discussed.

Further studies

After you have dealt with your findings in relation to previous work and any clinical or scientific implications, you are ready to suggest further work in the area. Some editors dislike the speculation that this entails and you may find that this paragraph(s) is subsequently deleted. For other research workers this is often the most interesting part of the discussion as it gives ideas for future research. However, before you parade your best ideas in public you are advised to have started the work otherwise you may find that other research groups publish first. If you do not intend to continue working in the area then this part of the discussion may be useful for claiming precedence of ideas.

Conclusion

It has been traditional to finish the discussion with a brief concluding paragraph which is a succinct résumé of the major findings. This is increasingly omitted, or deleted by the editor, as it often repeats information that has already appeared in the structured abstract, results and at the start of the discussion. Many authors still prefer to finish the discussion in this way but you need to ensure that it is not a direct repetition of previous parts of the manuscript.

Acknowledgements

Many journals expect the source of funding for the research and any conflict of interest to be given at the beginning of the paper, even the title page. If the instructions to the authors are not explicit about the matter then these should be stated clearly in the acknowledgements. Funding bodies must be listed and any commercial links given. If you are unsure whether the study could have been influenced by any current or previous commercial undertakings, then declare everything and let the editor decide what should be included.

You should also acknowledge any person who enabled the study to proceed, but did not achieve authorship (see Chapter 16, Richard Horton). For example, medical colleague, technician, research nurse and statistician, and permission to cite these people should be obtained before the paper is submitted. Do not use the acknowledgements to flatter colleagues, such as the head of the department.

Finally, sometimes assessors and editors feel that they have made a greater contribution to the final published manuscript than the authors and yet they are never acknowledged!

Chapter 6 **Titles, abstracts, and authors**

Fiona Moss

Introduction

Getting a paper published is one thing. Writing a paper that is a 'good read' requires additional skill and thought. Professional writers – for example, journalists who write for a living – write for readers. They want their message to get to as many people as possible. Many papers submitted to medical journals are dull, and, on first reading, it is not clear what they are about. Messages are difficult to find and the reader is challenged by dense writing. Only the truly determined – usually people in the same micro-field – make it through to the end. Many papers published in medical journals are read by very few people.

In modern times, a person's academic worth equates with the number of papers they have 'authored'. They are under pressure to publish, so that papers can be considered for research assessment exercises and academic preferment. Often, the number of papers published is considered more important than their quality, and no marks are awarded for clarity of writing. But editors are readers too. So, a well-written paper with a clear message is more likely to get through the editorial process than one that is equally worthy but dull and impenetrable.

Preparation of a research paper is not the same as writing a novel: it is not an exercise in creative writing. Conventions exist for describing the study design, results, and details of statistical analyses, and few ways exist to describe molecular structures or lung function tests. Nevertheless, within the limitations of the form, it is possible to write for the reader with clarity as well as accuracy and without burying the important messages in turgid, jargon-ridden prose. The use of a simple and straightforward style is essential, but being clear about what the paper is about comes first. So start by making sure that the title and abstract are compelling as well as accurate. Truthfully, many people will not read much else. And unless the title and the abstract can 'grab' the reader, they are unlikely to read on.

Titles (Box 6.1)

The title is important. Consider it as the signpost that tells the reader what your paper is about and encourages them to invest time in your paper. Titles must be functional, should be direct, and need not be dull. Use simple

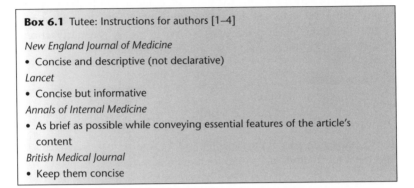

Box 6.1 Tutee: Instructions for authors [1–4]

New England Journal of Medicine
• Concise and descriptive (not declarative)

Lancet
• Concise but informative

Annals of Internal Medicine
• As brief as possible while conveying essential features of the article's content

British Medical Journal
• Keep them concise

language. Be concise, memorable, and informative, with an edge to alert the browsing reader and encourage them to read on, and with just enough detail for the focused reader to recognise the paper for which they have been searching (Box 6.2).

Box 6.2 Essential for titles

• Concise and precise
• Informative and descriptive
• Not misleading or unrepresentative
• Specific – for example, include type of study and numbers (if large)
• Words appropriate for classification
• Interesting not dull

Titles that are too clever or whimsical may briefly interest a browser but be missed by the purposeful reader. Avoid being very short and cryptic, as the words in the title may be used by electronic search engines to identify and categorise papers. To describe a comparative study of the prevalence of asthma in Birmingham and Hereford as 'A tale of two cities' would not work as a signpost for the reader and, given the binary logic of computers, might mean the paper is eventually linked electronically with papers on town planning.

Some tips (Box 6.3)

1 Describe your paper in two or three sentences.
2 Précis these sentences: remove unnecessary occurrences of 'as' and 'the', as well as any references to the results.
3 Now write a draft title.
4 Review this. Perhaps try the technique of 'a title in two parts', for example, giving the main subject and the type of the study. For example, 'Improving the repeat prescribing process in a busy general practice: a study using continuous quality improvement methods'.
5 Check:
   – Is it accurate?
   – Is it in any way misleading?
   – Does it contain essential key words?
   – Is it interesting?

It may be the only part of the paper that will be read, so make sure it encourages the reader to read on.

Box 6.3 Developing a title in four steps (after Lilleyman, 1998) [5]

1 An epidemiological geographically based study of the quantity and effects of ionising radiation received by male employees of a nuclear reprocessing plant and male residents working elsewhere in the same vicinity shows an increased risk of childhood leukaemia in the children of nuclear workers only.

2 An epidemiological study of the links between the radiation received by male employees of a nuclear reprocessing plant and other local residents and childhood leukaemia.

3 Relation between working at and living near a nuclear reprocessing plant and childhood leukaemia.

4 *'Nuclear reprocessing, radiation exposure, and childhood leukaemia: an epidemiological study'.*

Abstracts

Abstracts are usually the only part of the paper freely available via electronic search engines and are read by many more people than the rest of the paper. It is crucial, therefore, to sum up your paper in 200–300 words.

Structured abstracts are now the norm for papers that report original research. These provide a format that requires authors to summarise their work systematically by disclosing context, objectives, design, setting, participants, interventions, main outcome measures, results, and conclusions. Structured abstracts thus are informative and help peer reviewers and readers [6].

The abstract format is based on the standard IMRAD (Introduction, Methods, Results, And Discussion) structure of papers, but it is more detailed – for example, design, setting, participants, and interventions are sub-sections of the methods – so writing the abstract should ensure authors include essential detail in the main paper.

Abstract headings vary a little between journals and for different types of research. Not all research includes an intervention, and clinical research needs to describe participants, whereas meta-analyses include data sources and study selection. Unstructured abstracts are often required for papers that do not describe original research.

Structures based on the IMRAD format do not suit all types of work. Quality improvement work that includes repeated cycles of measurement and change cannot be easily expressed in the standard formats. To help authors express what matters in this type of work, the editorial team of *Quality and Safety in Health Care* devised a structure that reflects important aspects of quality improvement work [7,8]. The format includes, for example, strategies for change, lessons learned, and messages for others (see Box 6.4). Although the structure is different, the process and guidance for writing the abstract are the same.

Box 6.4 Structure for quality improvement reports

Context
- What are the relevant details of staff groups and functions of departments?

Outline of problem
- What were you trying to accomplish?

Key measures for improvement
- What would constitute success in the patient's view?

Process of gathering information
- What methods were used to assess problems?

Analysis and interpretation
- How did this information change your understanding of the problem?

Strategy for change
- What changes were made?
- How were they implemented?
- Who was involved?

Effects of change
- How did this lead to improvement for patients?

Next steps
- What have you learned/achieved?
- How will you take this forward?

Some tips

1 Start to write the paper by preparing the abstract. This may be the most difficult part of the paper to get right, but doing it first will help you to clarify your messages and make writing the rest of the paper easier.
2 Check:
   – Are abstract headings appropriate for the type of research?
   – Are they those required for the journal to which you are submitting: for example, background or context, objectives or aims, methods or design, results or outcome, and conclusions or discussion?
3 Check the maximum number of words. This varies between journals, but it usually ranges between 200 and 300 words.
4 Use phrases rather than sentences but maintain coherence and sense. Purple prose with too many adjectives and adjectival clauses has no place in scientific papers, but neither should the language be so terse that it becomes a knotted mass of words.
5 Check whether the abstract makes sense and that you are getting your message across. Ask a colleague who is not involved in the research to read it. Do they understand your message?
6 Check for consistency. The abstract should reflect the paper and describe your message succinctly and accurately. As soon as the paper is written, compare the abstract with the paper. Do the objectives described in the abstract match those in the paper? New words that change the emphasis can appear in the process of pruning for example appropriateness is not the same as suitability or usability.
7 Finally, remember that more people read the abstract than the whole paper and that many only read the abstract and may only give it one try.

Authors (or contributors?)

Authors are writers – at least that is the common usage of the word. Rohinton Mistry, Sara Paretsky, and JK Rowling are authors. They write. They create. The Harry Potter books – from idea to manuscript – are the work of JK Rowling. The word author also describes originators or creators other than writers, for example, the author of this plan or the author of congestion charging in London. When used in reference to papers in medical and scientific journals, however, the word author has a meaning that stretches beyond standard usage. Moreover, only rarely is there a single author of a medical paper. Authorship is shared with others. Clearly many authors are neither the originator nor the writer of the paper, but they are all essential to the team, to the development of ideas, to the technical input, and to the interpretation of results.

Authorship is a valued commodity that can be given and withdrawn. It can be 'gifted' in several ways. Firstly, 'back scratching' is when researchers working in related areas in the same unit swap authorships by putting each other on their papers, thus bolstering the number of papers that each has 'authored'. Secondly, 'toadying' is the custom of including, as authors, senior people who have influence but only a tenuous link to the paper – they may have been asked to look at an early draft, although they may not actually have read it. Thirdly, 'patronage' involves including as authors those involved solely because of routine administrative or technical tasks – usually, for example, seventh in a list of 10.

Less is known about the dark practice of not including people with a legitimate claim to authorship. Many stories exist, and are told and retold, of colleagues who, despite contributing hugely to all stages of a project, were dropped from the final list of authors. Radiologists regularly complain of being excluded from authorship of case reports that rely on radiographic findings or images. This isn't always dented pride: without their input, case reports sometimes wrongly describe findings.

Defining who should or should not be an author is not straightforward, and editors and researchers sometimes disagree. The Vancouver guidelines state that 'each author should have participated sufficiently in the work to take public responsibility for the content' and that authorship credit should be based on substantial contributions to:

1 concept and design or analysis and interpretation of data;
2 drafting of the article or revising it critically for important intellectual content;
3 final approval of the version to be published.

Authors must meet all three criteria. All other contributions, including data collection, should be mentioned in acknowledgements [9].

Editors, it seems, are less tolerant than researchers about including people who have contributed technically. Researchers do not like editors to make decisions about who or who should not be considered an author and although they may agree with each of the three 'Vancouver criteria', many are unhappy about having to meet all of them [10]. Much is at stake for researchers, because authorship is a sign of academic success.

Contributorship

Being an author gives credit, but it also carries responsibility. In some cases of publication of fraudulent data, co-authors have not accepted responsibility. The many problems with authorship – from gifting and ghosting to fraud and acceptance of responsibility – have led to the suggestion that authorship should be scrapped. Instead, people should be listed as contributors with a clear statement of each person's role, and, importantly, someone should take the role of guarantor of the paper [11–13].

That suggestion was first made in 1997. Authorship and debate about authorship continue, but several journals, including *JAMA*, *BMJ*, and *Lancet*, list each author's contribution. In addition, as one defence against publication of fraudulent work, some journals require one contributor to be identified as the guarantor responsible for the study. The Vancouver group recommends that the guarantor provides a written statement to acknowledge that they accept responsibility for conduct of the study, that they had access to data, and that they controlled the decision to publish.

Conventions of order

The Vancouver guidelines suggest that nothing should be inferred from the order of authors (because conventions between countries, specialties, and research groups differ). Much is assumed, however, and the position of first author is coveted [14]. If more than six authors are involved, many journals include the first three and sum up the rest as '*et al.*' The first author is likely to have been the person who wrote the paper, and the second and third authors are likely to be significant contributors. The last author is usually the heavy weight and is likely to be the guarantor – but not always, hence the need for the clarification provided by contributor lists.

Some tips

- Discuss 'contributorship' early on.
- Ask everyone to write down their contribution.
- Agree contributions.
- Establish who is to be guarantor.
- Ensure that all contributors can see raw data.
- Arrange for all contributors to meet to discuss interpretation of data.
- Ensure that all contributors have the opportunity to comment as the paper is drafted.
- Agree order of contributors.
- Agree who should be acknowledged.

References

1 *BMJ* house style. http://bmj.com/advice/stylebook/start.shtml
2 http://www.annals.org/shared/manu format.html
3 http://www.thelancet.com/
4 Help for Authors. http://www.neim.org/hfa/

5 Lilleyman JS. Titles, abstracts, authors. In: *How to Write a Paper*, 2nd edn. London: BMJ Publishing Group, 1998.

6 Haynes RB, Mulrow CD, Huth EJ, Altman DG, Gardner MJ. More informative abstracts revisited. *Ann Intern Med* 1990;**113**:69–76.

7 Moss F, Thomson R. A new structure for quality improvement reports. *Qual Saf Health Care* 1999;**8**:76.

8 Smith R. Quality improvement reports: a new kind of article. *BMJ* 2000;**321**:1428–9.

9 Uniform requirements for manuscripts to medical journals. http://www.icmie.org/

10 Bhopal R, Rankin J, McColl E, *et al.* The vexed question of authorship: views of researchers in a British medical faculty. *BMJ* 1997;**314**:1009–12.

11 Rennie D, Yank V, Emanuel L. When authorship fails: a proposal to make contributors accountable. *JAMA* 1997;**278**:579–85.

12 Smith R. Authorship is dying: long live contributorship. *BMJ* 1997;**315**:696.

13 Horton R. The signature of responsibility. *Lancet* 1997;**350**:5–6.

14 Chambers R, Boath E, Chambers S. The A–Z of authorship: analysis of influence of initial letter of surname on order of authorship. *BMJ* 2001;**323**:1460–1.

Chapter 7 **References**

Simon Howell and Liz Neilly

Introduction

The references of your paper are the foundation on which your work is built. They provide the scientific background that justifies the research you have undertaken and the methods you have used. They provide the context in which your research should be interpreted. They should not be collected as an afterthought when your research project is complete. A literature search and reading of the relevant references should be the starting points of any research project. Undertaking research to confirm the findings of another study of course is entirely justified. It is futile, however, to invest many hours of time and effort in a research project, only to discover that your findings are well-established facts that have been confirmed in many previous studies. In some cases, such a study could be argued to be unethical, in that it subjects animals, volunteers, or patients to research that leads to no new knowledge or understanding.

Searching the literature

The advent of electronic bibliographic databases of the medical and scientific literature has transformed the exercise of performing a literature search. These databases are generally accessible via the Internet and have stored within them the details of many thousands of references from hundreds of journals. The records are usually indexed in various ways to facilitate searching and provide tools that allow simple and more sophisticated interrogation of the database. A search that previously would have required many hours in a library ploughing through the large volumes of the *Index Medicus* can now be completed in a few minutes sitting at a computer. The speed and range of these electronic tools is such, however, that the searchers may find themselves swamped by an avalanche of citations. Some thought and practice is needed to get the best from these powerful tools.

Many bibliographic databases cover various aspects of the medical and scientific literature and may be relevant to the medical researcher. Probably the two most widely used are Medline and EMBASE. Medline is produced by the United States National Library of Medicine and covers the fields of medicine, nursing, dentistry, veterinary medicine, the healthcare system, and the preclinical sciences. It contains over 11 million citations that date back to the mid-1960s. EMBASE, the Excerpta Medica database, is produced by Elsevier Science. About 30% of journals that may be searched through EMBASE also appear in Medline, but EMBASE has a more European emphasis than Medline and is useful for identifying citations in non-English language journals. EMBASE has a strong emphasis on drugs, pharmacology, and toxicology, and it is particularly valuable for identifying citations in these areas. To complete a comprehensive search, you need to examine both databases. For clinical research, and especially for those planning a clinical trial or systematic review, a visit to the Cochrane Library (http://www.the-cochranelibrary.com) is essential. At the core of the Cochrane Library is its database of systematic reviews. It also contains a number of other valuable resources, including its Clinical Trials and Methods Studies databases.

A large number of other databases are available (Box 7.1). Among these, CINAHL covers the nursing and allied health literature, PsycINFO is a useful

---

Box 7.1 Common databases

Allied and Complementary Medicine Database (AMED)
Applied Social Sciences Index and Abstracts (ASSIA)
British Nursing Index (BNI)
Cumulative Index to Nursing and Allied Health Literature (CINAHL)
Digital Dissertations
Health Management Information Consortium Databases (HMIC)
National Research Register (NRR) (an NHS research register)
Popline (a population database)
PsycINFO (database of psychological abstracts)
Sociological Abstracts
Toxline (bibliographic database for toxicology)

---

gateway to the psychological and psychiatric literature and HMIC is a valuable resource for research in health management. It is easy to be overwhelmed by the extent and complexity of what is available. Start by searching the 'mainstream' databases discussed above and, if you find it is essential to venture more widely, seek the advice of a medical librarian. They will be able to tell you what databases are available locally, which may be relevant, and how best to search them.

The various databases have a number of different search interfaces. Among the most widely used are PubMed and Ovid. The former gives access to a free, easy search version of the Medline database via a service maintained by the United States National Library of Medicine. It can be found at http://www.ncbi.nlm.nih.gov/entrez. Although PubMed is freely available on the Internet and has a more user friendly interface than Ovid, it only provides access to one bibliographic database. In contrast, Ovid is a commercial organisation that provides access to a wide range of bibliographic databases including Medline and EMBASE. The precise databases available via Ovid vary according to subscriptions arranged by your institution. The Ovid user interface is more complex than that provided by PubMed, but it is a more powerful tool for complex searches. Ovid also has the merit that it includes a range of other databases for searching, in addition to Medline and EMBASE. Ask your local medical library for details of which databases are available and how to access them.

To conduct basic searches with these databases is not difficult. The user is provided with a box into which to type keywords, authors' names, or the title of a journal. Such a query may produce the response that no matches were found, but more frequently, a list of citations is returned. This may be several hundred references in length and could include material that is highly relevant, as well as citations that are not relevant at all. For this reason, you should gain some skill in searching these databases, as time invested in doing this will be repaid many times over in the future. Ovid provides extensive help files that explain how to get the best from the search engine. PubMed has help files and an extremely good interactive tutorial that provides an excellent introduction to how to use the database. Training and support may also be available from your local medical library.

All entries in Medline are indexed with a detailed set of medical subject headings or 'MeSH' terms – over 15 000 of which cover the whole range of medical subjects. Most MeSH terms have associated subheadings which can be used to focus on areas of special interest within your search topic, such as epidemiology or therapeutics. A search using MeSH terms is likely to be more successful and comprehensive than a general keyword query. PubMed provides a browser of MeSH terms, so you can identify and use the relevant terms. In Ovid, the 'mapping' function helps the user locate the most appropriate heading(s). EMBASE uses a similar set of subject headings, which may again be accessed using the mapping facility provided by Ovid. If you are unsure of the relevant MeSH terms or subject headings for your search, use the database to identify a reference you know to be relevant, look inside the record at the MeSH field and note the terms used to index that reference. You can then build those headings into your own search to develop your strategy.

Both Ovid and PubMed allow the history of the current search strategy to be examined and the search to be refined. The 'My NCBI' facility in PubMed and the 'Save search/alert' facility of Ovid allow details of the search to be saved, so it can be run again at a later date. Other tools allow limits to be set on what citations are returned by a given search: for example, a date range can be specified, the type of reference to be returned can be selected (e.g. review or randomised controlled trial), studies of animals or of humans may be requested, and the search may be limited to English language references only.

A particularly useful feature of these databases is the facility that allows searchers to find references that cover the same material as a given citation. Beside each reference identified in a PubMed search is a link labelled 'Related articles'. Clicking this link initiates a search that identifies references that cover similar material to the original citation. In Ovid, the same feature is available and is called 'Find similar'. Ovid also enables the user to locate references that have cited the original paper – this is performed using the appropriate 'Find citing articles' link.

Apart from a formal search strategy with medical subject headings, often it is useful to search for papers written by known workers in the field of interest. When you identify references through Medline, you may discover that, in some cases, the title carries the suffix 'see comment' and links to correspondence about the paper. Such correspondence may offer useful pointers to the interpretation of the paper and may be an indicator of current debate in the field of interest.

In both Ovid and PubMed, the abstracts of the references found can be displayed (where available). You should scan these online and select relevant ones to download and print. (The alternative is to print the references and read them offline, but you could end up printing out an unconscionably large number of references.) The 'clipboard' facility of PubMed allows selected references to be stored online, while further searches are conducted. The results of these further searches can be added to the clipboard, the contents of which can be downloaded and printed when searching is complete. Both PubMed and Ovid offer the facility to view, save, and print results as a text file rather than in hypertext mark up language (HTML) format. Printing in text format saves a considerable amount of paper. Apart from saving and printing text files, you may also wish to save references in a format that can be exported to reference management software. This is discussed further below.

Although bibliographic databases are immensely powerful, they are not the only source of relevant articles. Many journals are now available electronically, and you may search journals in the area of interest online for relevant material. A number of journals, including the *BMJ* (http://www.bmj.com/collections/) and the *New England Journal of Medicine* (http://content.nejm.org/collections/), have electronic archives of previously published papers and reviews, which are organised by subject. Finally, do not neglect the citations in the reference lists of the relevant papers and reviews that you find.

After you have completed your initial literature search and identified relevant references, obtain and read the papers. The abstract of a paper should be an accurate rendition of the contents of the paper, but this is not always the case. A study, originally published electronically and described subsequently in New Scientist, modelled the way in which errors in citations spread through the literature [1,2]. The study suggested that 78% of citations are 'cut and pasted' from a secondary source. The only way to be sure of what a paper says is to read it!

You may find that, no matter how focused you make your bibliographic search, you end up with an unmanageably large number of references. In this case, reading one or two good review articles may provide a gateway to the literature, by explaining the direction of current thought and placing the references you have found in context. If a carefully conducted search yields a large number of references, however, this often indicates that your field of interest is complex and researched widely. It is always wise to seek the advice and support of experts before embarking on new research. If the relevant literature is extensive, expert help is essential.

Managing references

You will find that it does not take long to accumulate a considerable number of paper references. Although storing these in a pile on the corner of your desk keeps them accessible, sooner or later this system will become unmanageable, and your references will start to find their way mysteriously into other piles of paper, on to the floor, and even into the waste bin. Few things are more frustrating than being unable to find a reference that took 2 weeks to arrive through an interlibrary loan. Devise some simple system for filing and retrieving your papers. I store papers in alphabetical order by the name of the first author. An alternative system involves numbering and storing papers sequentially, and keeping a record of the number in an alphabetical card index or in the database of an electronic reference manager (see below).

Considerably more is involved in managing references than simply keeping track of the paper copies, however. You need to know the relevance of each reference, which references you have cited in your manuscript and the order in which these references come together to form the bibliography of your paper. Traditionally, writers and researchers have done this using a card index system. Each reference is given a numbered index card and the numbers on these cards can be used to indicate citations in a manuscript and to bring together the references for the final bibliography. This system works well, but is labour intensive, and it can become cumbersome when managing a large number of references. The task has been much simplified by the advent of reference management software. A number of different software titles are available; the two most commonly used products are EndNote and Reference Manager – both of which are produced by Thomson ResearchSoft.

When you choose which product to use, you should ensure that it is compatible with your word processing software, so that the reference management software and word processor work together to allow you to insert citations in the text and produce a bibliography. You should also be able to import citations from EMBASE, PubMed, and other databases into your reference management database. These and other tasks are discussed in more detail below. It is often wise to find out which products colleagues use, as they may be able to offer help and support. Local support and licensing arrangements may be available for one or another product.

Reference management software

An electronic reference manager is basically an electronic database that has been adapted to a particular task. It allows you to build up and work with a personal library of references, and this library is therefore at the core of the product. You should be able to view a list of the references that you have stored, sort them by various criteria (such as first author or year of publication), and search them by various criteria. Most reference managers provide a notes section within each reference, into which you can type your own notes as to the relevance and importance of the reference.

One of the great benefits with this software is that references can be imported directly into the reference manager rather than having to be typed in by hand. Most reference managers can recognise and import a variety of different reference formats. The reference or references to be imported are identified in a bibliographic database, or other compatible electronic source, and are displayed and saved in an importable format. In this format, each field is given a tag that allows it to be identified by other programmes (e.g. AU for author and TI for title). The reference manager software is then instructed to import the references from the saved file with the appropriate import format – for example, 'Medline' for references saved from the Medline database. In this way, references may be added to your own library with the minimum of effort and a smaller chance of error than if the references were typed in by hand.

Despite the ease of this process, you need to be aware of some pitfalls. It is easy to import the same reference on a number of different occasions and hence end up with several duplicate copies in your library. Check that the authors of each reference are given correctly. If a committee prepared the paper or review, it may be listed in Medline as having no authors. Be aware that the title of the reference given in Medline may carry the suffix 'see comment', which refers you to correspondence about the paper. This will have to be removed in your reference manager database before the reference can be exported to your final bibliography. The journal title may be abbreviated, and both the full title and conventional abbreviations may have to be entered into the journals section of your reference manager. Finally, beware the temptation to transfer every reference that you find into your library. Enter only relevant and useful references, because there is no point storing citations that you may never look at again. Databases such as Medline and EMBASE exist to allow you to find such references when you need them.

Referencing your paper

After you have completed your literature search, designed your study, obtained ethical approval, and completed your research, you will finally have reached the stage of writing. In your manuscript, you will need to refer to the works of those who have gone before or perhaps to your own previous research in this field; placing markers in the text that refer the reader to references cited in the reference list or bibliography at the end of your paper. Some of your citations will appear in the introduction to explain why you have undertaken the research, and some may have a place in the methods section to justify and support the methods you have used, but most almost certainly will belong in the discussion, where you seek to explain and interpret your results. You must be selective in your use of references. Most journals limit the number of references that may be appended to a paper. Certainly, no editor will welcome a 1500 words manuscript with 60 references attached. On the other hand, you should cite such material as is necessary to support your work and attempt to produce an inclusive discussion that acknowledges viewpoints other than your own.

It is in the task of referencing a manuscript that reference management software comes into its own. If you use the index card system, each citation has to be marked on the manuscript with an index card number and, when the manuscript is complete, all of the citations have to be collated by hand and a final reference list typed up. An electronic reference manager greatly reduces both the labour involved and the opportunity for error. If the referees request the inclusion of extra references, these can be inserted and the reference list renumbered automatically. If your manuscript, unfortunately, is rejected by one journal and you need to reformat it for submission to another, such reformatting can be done quickly and easily by the software.

The reference management software and word processor are run in parallel. When the need to cite a reference or references arises, these are highlighted in the reference manager database, and, with the click of a mouse, unique identifiers for the references are pasted into the text. When the manuscript is complete, the reference manager is instructed to produce a formatted bibliography. The reference manager replaces each citation in the text with an appropriate reference number (Vancouver and related styles) or the name of the first author (Harvard and related styles), and an appropriately formatted reference list is appended to your document. In many programmes, your original file will be overwritten by the new version, so take care to save your original manuscript under a new file name before using the format bibliography command. If you have not kept a version with the citation markers in the text, when the time comes to make corrections to your paper, you may have to go through the manuscript and insert the markers all over again.

Reference formats

Two main formats exist for referencing papers: the Vancouver and the Harvard formats. The former increasingly is preferred for scientific literature. It arose from an informal meeting of a group of editors of medical journals held in Vancouver in 1978. The requirements for manuscripts laid down by the Vancouver group were first published in 1979. The Uniform Requirements for Manuscripts Submitted to Biomedical Journals, as these guidelines have become known, have been through a number of revisions, and journals are now asked to cite a version published in 1997 or later in their instructions to authors [3,4].

In the Vancouver format, references are numbered consecutively as they appear in the text and are identified by Arabic numerals in brackets. (Some journals require a different arrangement for review articles, in which the references are arranged alphabetically in the bibliography and numbered accordingly in the text.) In the Harvard system, references are cited in the text by giving the name of the author and the year of the publication in brackets. When a number of references are given together, they should be listed in chronological order separated by semicolons. In the bibliography, the references are listed in alphabetical order by author.

In your manuscript, the reference list at the end of the paper should begin on a new sheet of paper. The fine details of how references should be presented vary from journal to journal, and you should be sure to read the instructions for authors and examine the reference format for the journal to which you plan to submit your manuscript. Many of the reference manager software packages have built into them routines to produce bibliographies for many of the main journals. The usual conventions for the most common forms of citation are given below. Conventions also exist for referencing theses, conference proceedings, and web pages.

Journal article
Surnames and initials of authors. Full title of paper. *Title of Journal.* Year of publication; **Volume number:** First and last page numbers of article.

Example
Nunn JF, Bergman NA, Coleman AJ. Factors influencing the arterial oxygen tension during anaesthesia with artificial ventilation. *British Journal of Anaesthesia.* 1965; **37:** 898–914.

Book or monograph
Surname and initials of authors. *Full title of book.* Number of edition. Town of publication: Publisher; Year of publication.

Example
Robinson PN, Hall GM. *How to Survive in Anaesthesia.* 2nd ed. London: BMJ Books; 2002.

Chapter in multi-author book
Chapter author (surnames and initials). Chapter title. In: Book authors or editors (surnames and initials). *Book title.* Town of publication: Publisher; Year of publication. First and last pages.

Example
Goodman NW. Evidence based medicine: cautions before using. In: Tramer M, editor. *Evidence Based Resource in Anaesthesia and Analgesia.* London: BMJ Books; 2000. pp. 3–22.

Conclusion

Preparation of the references for a paper takes care and organisation. It is not a task that should be neglected; rather the search for relevant references should be the starting point for any research project. Failure to conduct a proper literature search at the outset may lead to embarrassing and potentially serious oversights. It is important not only to obtain the relevant papers, but to read them! When the time to start writing comes, attention to detail in referencing your manuscript and preparing the bibliography is essential. Modern software aids have made the task of managing references much easier, but diligence and care are still necessary. Failure to present an accurate reference list looks sloppy and may encourage the manuscript's assessors to be more critical.

Finally, and perhaps most importantly, finding, reading, and understanding references can be onerous, but do not deny yourself the hidden intellectual pleasures that can come with the task. Discussing the 'state of the art' and the formulation of research questions with knowledgeable colleagues may lead you into some fascinating conversations. Furthermore, as time passes and your work progresses, you may come to realise that you have developed quite an authoritative understanding of the state of knowledge in your area of interest. These are quiet, but real, pleasures.

References

1 Simkin MV, Roychowdhury VP. *Read before you cite!* Available from: http://www.arxiv.org/abs/cond-mat/0212043.
2 Muir H. Misprinted citations finger scientists who fail to do their homework. *New Scientist* 2002;**176**:12.
3 International committee of medical editors. Uniform requirements for manuscripts submitted to biomedical journals. Available from: http://www.icmje.org.
4 International committee of medical editors. Uniform requirements for manuscripts submitted to biomedical journals. *Ann Intern Med* 1997;**126**:36–47.

Chapter 8 **Electronic submissions**

Natalie Davies

The Internet has revolutionised our lives completely over the past few years. We can do our grocery shopping, apply for a mortgage, book a holiday, and buy a car from Japan – all in a matter of minutes. We can search for any information we require, and it is ours at the touch of a button. Its time saving properties are unequalled. This revolution has also been transmuted into the medical community. Nearly all of the hundreds of traditional medical journals available have an online version that faithfully mirrors the print journal (and in some cases improves upon it). More and more researchers, academics, and clinicians are turning to the online version, because they know that they can access the information they require much more quickly than searching through piles of paper journals. We are now travelling at an even greater speed down the 'information superhighway'.

Although revolutionising the lives of consumers, the impact the Internet has had on information suppliers, and in this case medical publishers, has been immense. Since the publication of the second edition of this book in 1998, much has changed within medical journal publishing. Maurice Long's chapter, 'The future: electronic publishing' foretold some of these changes – notably that 'more and more communication between authors, referees, publishers, and readers will be conducted over the net' [1]. In the years since the publication of Long's chapter, this prediction has come to pass for nearly all medical publications.

Electronic submission is not new. The medical community expects the dissemination of research to be speedier than ever before, while still being able to rely on the accuracy of the data. Consequently, authors have demanded that publishers speed up the peer review process and provide quick decisions on papers. This demand has led many journals to utilise the large number of electronic tools available to try and make the peer review process more efficient. Thus, what began as asking for manuscripts to be submitted as electronic copy on disc, progressed to asking for manuscripts to be submitted via email. The next logical step was to use the Internet for the submission and review of manuscripts.

Publisher's perspective

At the BMJ Publishing Group, we first began to research the possibility of implementing a web-based system in 1999. This was mainly because of the points outlined above, as well as an additional cry from our editors. After evaluating the systems available and testing two of them on two of our journals, we elected to adopt Bench>Press (by HighWire Press) as our system of choice. All the systems available are reasonably similar in construct,

---

Box 8.1 Guidelines for author submission

Please note: terminology and required items may be slightly different depending on the system the journal uses. The terms are usually similar and easily identifiable, however, and the individual journal's 'Instructions for authors' should always be read before submission.

1 Access the website via the URL by using a unique user identifier and password.
2 Enter the author submission area.
3 Choose the 'Submit a new manuscript' link.
4 Enter the manuscript meta-data. This usually consists of the following basic information: number of authors, type of article, title, manuscript keywords, abstract, cover letter to the editors, author details, suggested reviewers' names, and word count. Most journals ask for extra information, but this is usually explained in the instructions for authors and on the submission pages.
5 Enter the number of files you are uploading. This consists of one file for the actual article plus the number of image files associated with the manuscript.
6 Search on your computer for your manuscript files and enter the pathway into the appropriate field (e.g.: C:/My documents/Manuscript title).
7 Follow the system's guidance to 'upload' the article to the website.
8 The article is converted automatically into a pdf. This is mainly for reviewing purposes and accessibility issues. The pdf file size is smaller than standard word processing and image files, and the software required to view it (Acrobat Reader) is a standard piece of software easily obtained free of charge from the web (http://www.adobe.com).
9 You then have the opportunity to view your submission before it is submitted formally to the journal. This allows you to make sure that what you are submitting is correct and of peer review standard.
10 Once approved, the article is then considered to be a formal submission.

allowing authors to use different systems quite painlessly; however, Bench> Press suited our needs better than some of the other systems on the market. An intensive evaluation and implementation programme followed, which was finally completed in October 2002. All BMJ journals now use Bench> Press.

What does web submission mean?

In its simplest form, a web-based submission and review system is a database held on a website and accessed via a unique address (URL). This allows authors to access the database from any computer that has access to the Internet: whether in the office or home, at a conference centre, or even at a hotel. Authors enter the website, complete a series of fields, upload their manuscript to the database, and *voilà*, the manuscript has been submitted to the journal (see Box 8.1 for detailed author submission guidelines). The old adage of 'the manuscript was lost in the post' can no longer be applied. This is not the end of the story, however. Nearly all web-based systems in use by publishers offer a fully integrated system that means the *whole* peer review process is also conducted via the website.

What happens to the article once it has been submitted?

In the traditional manuscript submission process, authors would submit three or four hard copies of the paper to the editorial office. These would be logged on to a computer, and a copy would be passed to the editor (who is quite often based in a different building, town, or even country) for evaluation. The editor then decided if the manuscript was suitable for the journal and sent his or her decision to the editorial office for action. If the article was considered suitable, it would be posted to suggested reviewers and would then be filed until the reviewers' comments were received. On receipt of the comments, the manuscript again would be posted to the editors for an initial decision. The decision would be made and sent to the editorial office, and a letter posted to the authors. If the initial decision asked the authors to revise their article and resubmit, the manuscript would enter the cycle again. As you can imagine (and may have experienced), this could take an inordinate amount of time. On average, authors could expect to receive an initial decision within 12 weeks, and this does not take into consideration the time taken by those journals that discuss papers with all the editors of the journal at an editorial committee.

Using the web removes many of the above steps. The new Internet-based systems in place now enable the peer review process to be more streamlined.

- Authors submit their manuscripts online, entering the meta-data traditionally entered by the journal's staff. The manuscript is automatically assigned an identification number, and is entered into the database, from where it is immediately available to editors.
- The editor views the manuscript online and makes an immediate decision or suggests peer reviewers.
- Staff contact the peer reviewers through the web system to ask if they are willing to review the article.
- Reviewers access the reviewers' area of the website and review the paper, submitting their comments via an electronic review form available online.
- Once all comments have been received, the paper and comments are immediately available to the editors, ready for them to make a decision.
- The editor's decision is emailed to the corresponding author.

The above steps show a simplified process, but the benefits the web has brought are obvious. However, authors can gain much more from web submission than purely a reduction in the all-important turnaround times, however.

Benefits of author submission

The benefits to authors are numerous. Not only have the delays inherent in the postal system been made redundant – particularly appreciated by those authors who submit from different countries – but the peer review process has also been made more transparent to authors. Previously, once authors had submitted their manuscript to the journal, they had no way of knowing what was happening until a decision was posted to them by the editors. By accessing the website, authors can now track their paper and see where it is at any given stage; the system allows authors to interact with the process.

Author benefits

1 *Removing the need for 'snail mail'*: Manuscripts can no longer be lost or delayed in the post. Authors (or their departments) no longer have the expense of posting three or four hardcopies of the article, which saves on paper, printer cartridges, photographic paper, envelopes, and postage costs.

2 *Approving the article*: Authors can carry out a final check of the paper before submission and correct any mistakes before it is considered. This is important, as some journals do return papers to authors if there is an omission or error, which causes further delays.

3 *Linked references*: Some systems will convert the references of the manuscripts into hyperlinks to Medline or the abstract or full text of the online

article (if hosted by HighWire Press). The system also hyperlinks the author's details to all previously published papers. This is an invaluable feature and is much appreciated by editors and reviewers. Please note that the references must be in the exact format specified by the journal for optimum linkage. Non-standard journal citations are also difficult to convert.

4 *Supplemental data*: Most web-based systems allow authors to upload supplemental data as well as the article and images. This can be anything from appendices, published articles, questionnaires, and extraneous data.

5 *Interrogation of the system*: Most systems allow authors to view the status of their article as it moves through the peer review process. This provides authors with an easy way to check on the progress of their article, for example, 'with editor for decision', 'with reviewers awaiting comments', etc.

6 *Contacting the journal*: Email links available throughout the system give authors an easy opportunity to contact journal staff for assistance.

7 *Reviewer's comments available online*: As soon as the editor sends a decision, the reviewer's comments are available online to authors.

8 *Author history*: Authors retain a record on the system of all manuscripts submitted to the journal, including the article itself, the editor's decision letter, and reviewer's comments.

9 *Personal information*: Authors can update their personal details and expertise terms at any time.

10 *Reduced turnaround times*: Perhaps most importantly, turnaround times can be dramatically reduced. At the BMJ Publishing Group, we have seen up to a 50% reduction in time taken to first decision.

Important points to remember

Although most web-based systems are reasonably self-explanatory, errors do sometimes occur. This is usually because authors have not properly read the journal's instructions for submission. It is imperative that the instructions are read before submission, as they often contain essential journal requirements as well as guidance on submission. This is particularly important when dealing with images. Most journals and/or web-based systems have strict instructions with respect to the format of image files, and it is essential that these are followed. Most systems in use accept the standard graphic formats: tif, jpg, gif, and eps, and usually there will be no problems with these. If in any doubt, contact the journal's office before submission. Other important points to take note of are:

• Always read the instructions for authors before submission and take careful note of journal requirements.

- All systems adopt a strict security system that is based on a user identification (unique email address or other identifier) and password system. This prevents unauthorised access to manuscripts and personal information, and it allows authors to track their manuscript through the process.
- Some systems encrypt passwords for further security and cannot be obtained by journal staff or the software suppliers. In these cases, a 'password hint' question and answer system is adopted.
- If the manuscript is accepted, the original word processing and image files (source files) may be requested if the files uploaded to the web-based system are not suitable for publication.
- If in any doubt, contact the staff of the editorial office, who will always be happy to help.

The future

The adoption of an electronic submission and peer review system may well help reduce the time from submission to decision; however, we are still living in a largely print-based world. The time from acceptance to publication can still be lengthy, and many journals have to limit the length of articles because of page restrictions. Many publishers are now starting to scrutinise this end of the process and to utilise the myriad benefits of the Internet to provide improvements. Such innovations include:

- publish ahead of print: articles are published online before publication in the print journal – in some cases, this can be some months in advance;
- publish online instead of in print;
- e-letters: authors can post immediate responses to published articles online;
- 'short' versions of the paper in print, with a longer, more detailed version online.

Many journals are also beginning to offer added 'web' benefits, including movies, extra images, data supplements, presentations, coming events, email alerts, cite track (this allows the author to track topics and authors in any of the participating journals), journal announcements, enhanced searching and display across topics and journals, course material, interactive educational material, and the facility to download articles to a personal digital assistant (PDA).

From the innovations listed above, the future may already seem to be here. Not so. New technologies are being developed quicker than ever. Medicine is constantly evolving. Our authors' and readers' needs change.

All of the innovations already in place are there in response to our authors' requirements. As such, everyone involved in the medical community – authors, reviewers, editors, readers, as well as publishers – can expect an exciting few years ahead!

Reference

1 Long M. The Future: Electronic Publishing. In: Hall GM, ed. *How to Write a Paper*, 2nd edn. London: BMJ Publishing Group, 1998, pp. 132–7.

Chapter 9 **How to write a letter**

Michael Doherty

General considerations

When you think of submitting a letter to a journal, first consider the following basic questions:

- What is the purpose of your letter?
- Is a letter format appropriate for this particular journal?
- Does what you want to say justify a communication?

The purpose of a letter varies between journals (Box 9.1). Most letters are comments in response to a previous publication, although brief communications that do not justify an extended or concise report are sometimes appropriate as letters. It is always wise to read the 'Instructions for authors' and to examine the correspondence section of recent issues of the journal to gain a feel for

---

Box 9.1 The purpose of a letter

Usual
- Comment (positive or negative) in response to a previous publication
- Concise communication of clinical or investigative data
- Communication of case report(s)

Less common
- General medical or political comment (e.g. 'guild issues')
- Comment concerning the nature or format of the journal
- Advertisement of interest to collaborate or to gain access to patients or study material

---

the style and scope of successful (i.e. published!) letters. Because the amount of information provided in a letter is necessarily limited, rarely is there justification for a long list of authors. Always question whether the information you wish to convey truly justifies publication – minor comments or observations are unlikely to be accepted.

If the purpose and content of your communication seem appropriate as a letter, two other major considerations are its length and the style of presentation. With respect to length, always be brief. Editors like concise communications. They would rather publish 10 short letters on 10 different topics than two lengthy ones on only two topics. Think how you react as a reader – messages are always more effective if put succinctly. Some journals impose firm restrictions on word count, number of references, and use of accompanying tables or figures, and these restrictions will be outlined in their instructions to authors. Even if not overtly stated, however, all editors favour a 'Raymond Chandler' over a 'Charles Dickens'. For example, compare the following two introductory paragraphs to the same letter.

Sir,

I feel I must put pen to paper with respect to the recent communication by Dr Peter Jones and colleagues in your August issue,[1] to draw the attention of your readers to possible misinterpretation of the data that they present. Although these excellent workers have an internationally renowned track record in the field of complement activation (not only in rheumatoid arthritis but in other inflammatory diseases as well), in this present study, they seem to have omitted to properly control for the varying degrees of inflammation in the knee joints of the patients that they aspirated – not only those with rheumatoid arthritis but also those with osteoarthritis. Such inflammation of the knee joint could have been assessed readily either by local examination and scoring of features such as temperature increase, effusion, synovial thickening, anterior joint line tenderness, duration of early morning stiffness, and the duration of inactivity stiffness, with addition of the different scores to a single numerical value (that is, the system devised and tested by Robin Cooke and colleagues in Alberta[2]) and/or by simultaneous measurement and comparison to levels of other markers of inflammation, for example, the synovial fluid total white cell and differential (particularly polymorphonuclear cell) count or local synovial fluid levels of various arachidonic acid products such as prostaglandins or leukotrienes ...

(Dr C Dickens)

Sir,

In their study of synovial fluid complement activation Jones *et al.*[1] made no assessment of the inflammatory state of aspirated knees. Such assessment could have been attempted using the summated six-point clinical scoring system of Cooke *et al.*[2] or by estimation of alternative indicators of inflammation (for example, cell counts, prostaglandins, or leukotrienes).

(Dr R Chandler)

Both convey the same message. The second is more 'punchy', however, and gets straight to the point by omitting unnecessary description and detail. As with any scientific writing, keep sentences short. Make each of your points separately. Reference short statements rather than provide extended summaries of previous work.

Etiquette and style for letters in response to an article

A letter is the accepted format for comment relating to a previous publication in the same journal. Occasionally it may relate to a publication in another journal. Note that letters are always directed to the editor, never to the initial author. The editor in this situation is an impartial intermediary between authors, particularly those in potential conflict.

The usual purpose of a responding letter is to offer support or criticism (most commonly criticism) of the rationale, method, analysis, or conclusion of the previous study. If this is the case, make specific, reasoned criticisms or provide additional pertinent data to be considered in the topic under consideration (Box 9.2). Do not reiterate arguments already fully covered or referenced in the provoking publication. Your letter should raise new points that were not addressed adequately or should provide additional information that

---

Box 9.2 Guidelines for a letter in response to an article

- Be courteous and interested – not rude or dismissive
- Make specific rather than general comments
- Give reasoned argument, not biased opinion
- Do not repeat aspects already covered in the original article
- Introduce a different perspective or additional data to the topic
- Attempt to make only one or a very few specific points
- Be concise

supports or refutes the contentions of the other authors. However prestigious you may think yourself, merely offering your personal dissent or approval is not enough. You should use the letter to argue a reasoned perspective. It should not be a vehicle for biased opinion. Always be specific. General comments unsubstantiated by reasoned argument ('I think this a great publication' or 'I think it is rubbish') are unacceptable.

If you are offering criticism, always be professional and courteous – never rude, arrogant, or condescending. Apart from common decency to fellow investigators, politeness in correspondence will serve to enhance and safeguard whatever reputation you have. This is the same golden rule that applies to question time at oral presentations. No one likes a rude critic, even (or more especially) one who is right. A polite, understated question or comment inevitably has more critical impact than arrogant dismissal. For example, compare the following two styles of presentation. Both letters make the same points.

Sir,

I was greatly surprised that the paper on synovial fluid complement breakdown products (C3dg) by Jones *et al.* managed to get into your journal. Firstly, Jones *et al.*[1] obviously forgot to control for the inflammatory state of the knees that they aspirated, even though our group previously has drawn attention to the importance of this in any study of synovial fluid.[2] Secondly, they made no attempt to determine levels of C3dg in synovial fluid from normal knees. Since they only compared findings between knees of patients with either rheumatoid or pyrophosphate arthritis, it is hardly surprising that they jump to the wrong conclusion in stating that complement activation is not a prominent feature of pyrophosphate arthropathy. Thirdly, they only reported crude C3dg concentrations, with no correction for synovial fluid native C3 levels. If these investigators had only taken the time to read the existing literature, they would have realised that we previously have shown that such correction is of paramount importance for correct interpretation of C3dg data. That such a majorly flawed paper, which does not even reference our seminal work,[2] should be published at all – let alone as an extended paper – must seriously question the effectiveness of the peer review system that you operate.

(A Pratt)

Sir,

I was interested in the study of synovial fluid breakdown products (C3dg) by Jones *et al.*[1] in which they conclude, contrary to our previous report,[2] that complement activation is not a feature of chronic pyrophosphate arthropathy. Such discordance most likely relates to differences in clinical characterisation and expression of C3dg levels rather than to estimation of C3dg itself. Unlike Jones *et al.* we assessed and controlled for the inflammatory state of aspirated knees, included normal knees as a control group, and corrected for native C3 concentrations (expressed as a ratio C3dg/C3), as well as reporting C3dg concentrations. By employing these methods, we were able to demonstrate complement activation in clinically inflamed, but not quiescent, pyrophosphate arthritis knees. Such activation was less marked quantitatively than that observed in active rheumatoid knees. We would suggest that clinical assessment of inflammatory state, inclusion of normal knee controls, and correction for native C3 levels be considered in future studies of synovial fluid.

(A Diplomat)

Remember that the original authors will usually be invited to respond to your criticisms. It is much easier to respond to a rude than a polite letter, and even potentially damning points that you raise may get lost in the 'noise' of confrontation. For example, Dr Jones would be able to centre his reply to Dr Pratt's letter on the defence of the peer review system. He would be hard pressed, however, to sidestep the same specific criticisms levelled by Dr Diplomat. Furthermore, the original authors have the last word, and if your criticisms are misplaced (it happens!) you may not be given the opportunity to rescind before publication. You may then find yourself publicly ridiculed, appearing as a rude ignoramus rather than an interested and inquiring intellectual. For example:

Sir,

We are grateful to Dr Pratt for his comments. We in fact had carefully considered all the points he raises. Because all knees included in our study were clinically inflamed, the question of correcting for differing degrees of inflammation does not arise. We also considered aspiration of normal knees, but this was not approved by our research ethics committee. We included estimation of native C3 and expression of C3dg/C3 in our original manuscript. This made no difference to the results and, because the main thrust of our paper dealt with the method – not the demonstration – of C3 activation in rheumatoid knees (with original data on C4d and factor B activation), we were asked to delete these data by the expert reviewers. We of course were aware of the study by Dr Pratt and colleagues, but we were limited in the number of references we could include. We referred therefore to the first report of synovial fluid C3dg in normal, rheumatoid, and pyrophosphate arthritis knees by Earnest *et al.*[1] which predated that of Pratt *et al.* by six years.

Other forms of letter

In many journals, the correspondence section is an appropriate site for short reports that have a simple message but do not necessitate a full paper. This is particularly true if a study uses standard techniques that are readily referenced and require no detailed explanation.

Studies

Presentation of a study as a letter is rather similar to writing an extended abstract (Box 9.3). Normally there should be three clear divisions: an introduction relating the rationale and objectives of the study; a section stating the

---

Box 9.3 Presentation of a concise report as a letter

Introduce the topic
• Briefly explain rationale and objectives of study.
Present methods and results
• Reference methods as much as possible to reduce length of their description
• Include only essential data
• If possible present data in a table and/or figure.
Present conclusions
• Emphasise only one or a few major conclusions
• Place findings in context of previous literature
• Highlight caveats and strengths of the study
• Suggest future studies that are still required in this area.
Avoid extrapolating too far from data.
Avoid repetition of data or conclusions.
Be concise.

---

methods, analysis, and results; and, finally, a conclusion. The conclusion should assess the validity and importance of the findings in the context of other work, highlight the caveats and strengths of the study, and indicate the direction of future-related research. Unlike concise or extended reports, section headings are not enforced, and an abstract is unnecessary. Nevertheless, subheadings may be used to good effect and often assist the clarity of presentation.

Although often considered a 'second-rate' way of reporting data, a letter format is quite appropriate for brief reports and can still be prestigious, especially in high-impact journals. If you are presenting original data in a letter, carefully consider whether this will compromise subsequent publication of the same data in a more extended form. Remember that letters can be referenced and that 'redundant' or duplicate publications must be avoided.

Case reports

Case reports are often presented as letters. They are particularly suitable for single cases that do not justify a full or concise report. Some journals have no specific slot for case reports and publish all cases as letters. Most editors only publish cases that give novel insight into pathogenesis, diagnosis, or management. To report the sixth case of concurrence of two diseases in the same patient is of no scientific interest – only a formal study, not further case reports, can answer whether this is chance concurrence or a true association that may give clues relating to pathogenesis of either disease. As with short reports, cases are best divided into a brief introduction, a description of the case itself, and then a discussion of its interest, with no section headings. Be particularly careful not to repeat the same information by summarising the case at the beginning and the end. This is a common and easy mistake.

General or political comment

General or political comment occurs mainly in major weekly journals or in specialist journals that are the official outlet of learned societies. In this situation, humorous comments may be permitted. Humour is always risky, however – especially for an international audience with diverse perspectives on what, if anything, is funny. Letters may be used to advertise an interest in particular cases or investigational material for research purposes or a service on offer (e.g. DNA repository). Such advertisements should be very brief and are more usually found in a notes or news section.

Chapter 10 **How to prepare an abstract for a scientific meeting**

Robert N. Allan

Introduction

How could anyone insist that your work, which is at the forefront of scientific development and has consumed your life in recent years, should be minimised to the size of an abstract box? Pause, recover your equilibrium, and muster a little sympathy for the organisers of the meeting where you plan to present your original work.

The scientific programme will have been planned several years in advance. The lectures and symposia will have been agreed, the national and international speakers invited, and the venue selected. The programme will also include a limited number of spaces for presentation of abstracts, either as oral communications or posters.

Selection of abstracts

The number of abstracts submitted nearly always exceeds the number that can be included so that some sort of selection procedure must be adopted. A panel of reviewers, each an expert in their own field, is asked to assess each abstract. Each has a large number of abstracts to assess, so the time allocated to your own precious abstract may well be short. Furthermore, the secretariat organising the meeting will know that authors often ignore instructions and submit abstracts which are over length, illegible, incomplete, or late. They will be determined on this occasion only to consider abstracts that conform to the published guidelines. Be warned!

Online submission of abstracts

Online submission is now the norm. The website of the society organising the meeting will include detailed information, and many meetings have a site dedicated to preparation of abstracts. For example, the British Society of Gastroenterology's home page (http://www.bsg.org.uk) provides direct access to the meetings website. Click on 'abstracts' for online preparation and submission.

Guidelines for online submission

Specific guidelines must be followed – only use the specified area and include the title, list of authors, institution, and address. Do not modify the page setup with respect to dimensions or font (print) size. You must declare originality or previous publication.

Snail mail submissions

Guidelines

A few meetings still use postal submissions. The instructions may look (and usually are!) tedious, but they are designed to ensure high-quality reproduction of your work. Abstracts are no longer edited and typeset. For speed and efficiency abstracts will be reproduced exactly as they first appear. The abstract must therefore be typed within the prescribed area. An appropriate size typeface and a high-quality laser printer should be used to ensure good reproduction. Direct reproduction of the camera ready abstract will mean that any errors in spelling, grammar, or scientific fact will be reproduced exactly, so take care. Vain hopes that the photographic process might in some way enhance your abstract must be abandoned.

Send the appropriate number of copies. Anonymous copies – without the names of the author and the institution where the work was carried out – are often requested to ensure that the marking system is independent and fair. Make a careful note of the deadline – preparation of abstracts always takes longer than expected. Late entries or those not conforming to the guidelines may be rejected out of hand, without evaluation. The abstract form commonly includes a number of subject categories. Identify the most appropriate category for your work to ensure that the selected reviewer is an expert in your field. Mark whether the abstract will be presented as a poster or oral presentation. You must declare that the abstract is completely original or submit details if the abstract has been submitted to another meeting or for publication. Full information must be provided.

Preparation of the abstract

The abstract should be prepared with a number of headings – even though the headings themselves may eventually be deleted from the final text.

Title

The title is a concise summary of the abstract and must demonstrate that the work is important, relevant, and innovative. Define the key features of your work and link them together until the title effectively conveys that message.

Authors

Include authors who have really contributed to the work. It is assumed, if the abstract is accepted, that the first author will present the work. The author presenting the work must be identified. The name and address of the institution at which the work was carried out is included, with a contact email address. For example, your abstract may be selected for a plenary session, and the organisers will need to confirm that the presenter speaks fluent English and that the work is sufficiently important to include in the session.

Background

Start with a sentence or two that summarises previous work relevant to the presentation. Highlight any controversies that your work has helped to resolve.

Aims

What is the point of the study? What is the hypothesis that is being addressed? How is your work different from previous work? Is it useful, exciting, and worthwhile? Does it make a new and significant contribution? To encapsulate these ideas in a sentence or two takes time and practice.

Patients

If patients were studied, how were they selected? Did they give informed consent? Was the selection of patients random? Why were patients excluded? Confirm that ethical committee approval was obtained.

Methods

The techniques employed must be summarised and novel methods described in greater detail. Minimise the use of abbreviations, which may confuse the reader and assessor. Include the methods used to test for statistical significance.

Results

Data about patients should be described first, including the numbers studied, sex, age, distribution, and duration of followup. The key results should then be summarised, usually in four or five sentences that identify the positive features; ensure that any claims can be substantiated. Highlight new developments.

Discussion

What has the work added to the existing body of knowledge? In what way are these new findings important? Could the findings have occurred by chance or are they statistically significant?

Conclusions

Why is the work important? How might the work be developed further?

From draft to final version

The draft abstract is now complete. It will be hopelessly over length. To edit this information to an abstract of less than 200 words is a challenge. Delete any duplicated, superfluous, or irrelevant information. Can the same idea be conveyed in fewer words? If the abstract is still over length, what are the most important results? Can some points be omitted and only presented at the meeting?

It will take time and many drafts to produce the final version. Start early and aim to complete and submit the abstract well before the deadline. The abstract must summarise the work, but must also excite the reviewer in that 'brief moment of time' when your abstract is being assessed.

Reread the guidelines and ensure that you have conformed completely with the instructions. Circulate the draft abstract to your colleagues and obtain their approval before submission.

Final preparation

The abstract can now be completed and the final version prepared. Do not duplicate submissions – two or more abstracts that describe similar results from the same study are both likely to be rejected. Include an email address for future communication.

Outcome

In due course, you will hear the outcome of the assessment and experience the joy of acceptance or the depression of rejection. Few abstracts are outstanding, and few are awful. The marks for most abstracts hover around the mean and abstracts are either just accepted or just rejected. Temper the joy of acceptance with modesty. The depression of rejection can be minimised by knowing that the abstract was probably only just rejected.

Presenting the data

The accepted abstract has to be converted into an oral presentation or a poster – another exciting challenge. Submission of an abstract implies that one of the authors will present the paper or poster in person at the meeting. Late withdrawal of an abstract gives both the individual and their unit a bad name.

Conclusion

An abstract that effectively summarises your work clearly and concisely with an apparently effortless presentation can only be achieved with meticulous preparation. In doing so, however, you will share in the excitement of contributing at the forefront of new scientific developments.

Chapter 11 **How to write a case report**

Martin Neil Rossor

In the hierarchy of evidence-based medicine single anecdotal case reports are at the very bottom, and yet case reports can be the vehicle for novel observations be they associations of diseases, unusual presentations, side effects of therapeutic interventions or even rarely new diseases [1]. Although there is legitimate concern about the selectivity of reporting, case reports can generate hypotheses for subsequent systematic research leading to a more secure evidence base. Individual case reports can also be educational and thus illustrative of what may be already well known but often forgotten. The large capacity of online publishing and the introductions of new publishing models of open access and author pays make it likely that publication of case reports will increase rather than decrease.

For many clinicians the case report has been their first successful publication. The task of preparing a case report is often delegated by busy clinicians to a junior member of the team. Case reports are not easy to write but a well-written report can be a delight to read.

Why publish a case report?

Having been involved with a patient that you think may be the basis of a report, it is important to be clear why the case should be published. This will help structure the article, help you to target the journal and will be important to include in a cover letter to the editor. Listed below are some of the reasons for publishing a case report:

A very rare disease

Rarity is often cited in covering letters to journals as the reason for reporting a particular case. However, rarity *per se* is seldom of interest to editors. Gaining information and experience about rare diseases is often better served by a report on a series of cases together with a more extensive literature review. Two patients with a very rare disease as a case report would be of more value than a single case.

Associations of diseases
This is also a commonly stated reason for reporting a particular patient. However, the chance association of common or rare diseases is again of little interest. For associations to be of interest, they need either to generate hypotheses about underlying causation or the association of the two diseases has created a particular challenge in management or diagnosis.

Rare presentations of more common diseases
A very unusual or previously unreported presentation of a common disease is likely to be of interest and publishable. The challenge is to substantiate your diagnosis and to exclude other explanations or coexistent disease.

Reporting a particular outcome
Reporting unexpected outcomes can be valuable. For example, an unanticipated good prognosis of a fatal disease or an unexpected side effect of an intervention. Although the case reporting of new side effects provides a poor evidence base because of publication bias, it nevertheless points the way to more systematic investigation.

Outcome of a novel treatment
It is the selective reporting of individual patient's responses to an intervention that has given case reports a bad name in evidence-based medicine. Many journals will not consider single case reports of therapeutic interventions unless the outcome is so striking, for example treatment of a hitherto fatal disease, or unless there has been a placebo phase.

Mistakes and lessons
Many journals will publish case reports purely for educational purposes. Lessons learned need not relate to rarities and indeed are often more educational if the problem is likely to be encountered in every day practice.

A new disease?
This is perhaps the least likely basis for a case report but is a most compelling reason for publication. However, claims of precedence in case reports are often proved wrong.

Choosing your journal

Once you have decided what the main reason is for your case report, it is worth considering possible journals before starting writing. In many cases you will need to target a specialist journal. Journals may publish case reports under a number of headings rather than just case reports, for example as a letter, as a 'lesson of the week' or as a 'picture'. Read through published case reports in the journal and read the instructions to authors very carefully and follow them precisely. Journals will vary on their requirements for case reports but, as a general guide, around 1000 words is a common length with one or two figures or tables. Although there is an argument for standardising case reports, this has yet to be achieved [2].

The structure of the case report

Most journals will expect you to follow a standard format of abstract, introduction, the case report itself and then discussion and perhaps conclusion followed by the references. It is important to remember that whereas cases are examples of the disease, patients are persons.

Not all journals will require an abstract and this is often the most difficult to write. It may be easier to wait until the main body of the article has been written and may just be a very brief sentence to summarise what is being reported and why. If the case report is in the format of a letter, it will often start with 'we report a 38-year-old man with extremely rare case report syndrome …'

The introduction will need to say why the case is being reported, with a brief introductory background. Some authors will include here a brief literature search but this may be better dealt with in the discussion.

The common format of the clinical details is to provide the history with the presenting features, the past medical history, social history and family history together with drug history. This is then followed by the physical examination, investigations, the differential diagnosis and then the treatment and outcome. However, it is important to present the information chronologically and this should tell a story. One may therefore need to set the scene with the presenting features, the past medical history, social history and family history and then to detail the chronology which will inevitably intersperse symptoms, signs and investigation as the story unfolds. Remember to avoid jargon and if acronyms and abbreviations are used they should be explained in the text. Normal value of laboratory results should be provided except for the routine. Important negatives should be mentioned both in the history, the examination and the investigation but only if essential to the message.

It is important to anonymise the patient as far as possible but this can never be complete. Clearly names and initials must be avoided, although unrelated initials are widely used, especially in the neuropsychology literature where detailed study of a single patient may constitute a major research paper. Identification by coded initials helps cross-referencing if the patient is part of more than one paper. Non-essential personal details should be omitted.

A table of results can be helpful and pictures of clinical signs or radiology can be invaluable. The faces of patients can be digitally masked to help preserve anonymity. In some instances, recognisable pictures may be important and are acceptable, provided fully informed consent is obtained (see below).

The discussion should be used to clarify the key issues and this may be the best place to refer to other cases and a summary of the literature. However, the case report is not the vehicle for an extensive review of the literature. Where a literature search has been done the methodology should be briefly stated. The final message should be summarised and this is where the claim must have been substantiated.

If new to medical writing it is important to get advice early and particularly with respect to the key message and reason for writing the case report. It is valuable to get other people to read the article and often helpful if they have not been involved in the patient's care. It is very easy to overlook an important point because one is too close to the case.

Consent

You will need the consent of the patient to publish. This is essential and many journals will not even send your article out for review unless a consent form accompanies the article when submitted. Many journals will have their own consent form and, if not, you should create your own using one of the other journal templates as a guide. In Europe the EU privacy laws make it illegal to publish confidential information without consent whether this is in print or online. A common misconception is that if no photograph or personal details are provided then there is no need for consent. This is not true. It is extremely difficult to anonymise completely and indeed for an individual case report this is essentially impossible as the key features would be lost. It is important, therefore, to contact the patient at the earliest opportunity and to explain that one would hope to publish a case report. Once patients understand that they will not be referred to by name and personal details minimised, then consent is usually forthcoming. Clearly with photographs, particular care needs to be taken. It is good practice to give a copy of the final article to the patient and then one can be secure in the knowledge that consent has been fully informed and given.

A duty of confidentiality persists even if the patient has died and in these instances the next of kin should be contacted.

Occasionally it may be difficult to obtain consent because the patient was seen a number of years ago, as may well happen if one is reporting two instances of a particular disease and it may be many years between the two cases. Patients may also move away and die. Rarely publication can go ahead but certain criteria need to be met. First, publication should be in the public interest and if that cannot be met then one should not be writing the case history in the first place. Second, every effort should have been made to contact the individual or next of kin. Third, every effort should be made to anonymise the case report. Fourth, one should assure oneself that the average person in this situation would be unlikely to withhold consent.

One should also consider the assent to publish from other clinicians involved in the care of the patient. Often these will be co-authors. Certainly the agreement should be obtained from the main clinicians involved in the care of the patient and they should see a copy of the article before submission.

Authorship

Journals offer guidance on authorship. Merely having the patient under one's care does not justify authorship; there needs to be intellectual input into the case report itself. The many clinicians involved in the care of the patient can be acknowledged but be aware that some journals require a letter from those you acknowledge confirming their involvement and agreement to acknowledgement. It is important to avoid a football team of authors and indeed many journals will restrict the number of authors for letters, lessons of the week or pictures.

Submitting the article

Before submission, ensure again that you have all the appropriate consents and assents to publish. Ensure that all the instructions and guidelines on the journal webpage are followed, particularly with respect to length of article and numbers of figures and format. Do write a cover letter which journal editors find very helpful. This should be succinct and state why this case report is of particular interest.

Good luck!

References

1 Vandenbroucke JP. In defence of case reports and case series. *Ann Intern Med* 2001;**134**:330–4.
2 Sorinola O, Olufowobi O, Coomarasamy A, Khan KS. Instructions to authors for case reporting are limited: a review of a core journal list. *BMC Med Educ* 2004;**4**:4.

Chapter 12 **How to write a review**

Paul Glasziou

Before asking 'how' to do a review, it is wise to first ask 'why'. The main reason for doing a review is to provide a readable synthesis of the best of the current research literature on an important question or topic. This simple definition of a review contains the three crucial elements we will explore in detail in this chapter:

1 the question or questions addressed in the review;
2 the methods to find and select the best of the research relevant to answer those questions;
3 the methods to synthesise the disparate studies found.

Determining the important questions to answer usually requires some preliminary scoping of the literature, discussions with others in the field, and time spent in reflection. Tempting though it is to move on to writing the review, time spent clarifying which are the important questions is always time well spent [1]. Some tricks to doing this are asking 'why' five times: ask why is the answer to the question important (and why is that answer important, etc.). You might try also drawing a causal schema – an arrow diagram of the chains of causation – showing what are the causes and consequences of the problem addressed.

However, a review can never be 'complete' as questions are fractal: as we examine them there are further smaller questions that arise. For example, we can ask if cholesterol reduction reduces the risk of stroke, but then wonder about the many subgroups of patients, and many ways of lowering cholesterol, or the mechanism, or the duration of therapy needed, and so the list goes on. It is best to sketch out the broader scope, but then narrow down to the most crucial issues.

The content and format

Before we look at the writing process, it is worth understanding what a good review might look like. There are several varieties of review, each with a legitimate role, for example:

(i) The answer to a single focused question, such as, 'do statins reduce the risk of stroke?' or 'can raised b-natriuretic peptide accurately diagnose heart failure?'

(ii) An overview of several related single questions, such as 'which treatments can lower the risk of stroke' or 'what is the relative value of ECG, b-natriuretic peptide, and chest X-ray in the diagnosis of heart failure'.

(iii) A topic review, such as the diagnostic processes for specific conditions (the JAMA series on the Rational Clinical Examination are good examples of these [2,3]).

Whichever the type, an important distinction is between a systematic and a non-systematic review. The difference between these is largely in the methods used to identify the literature. A non-systematic review will use the papers that you happen to have collected over the years or that colleagues have mentioned, whereas a systematic review begins with the questions and then systematically searches for the best research available to answer those questions.

Unfortunately such a systematic process is not the norm: a check of reviews in six general medical journals in 1998 found that less than a quarter described how evidence was identified, evaluated, or integrated; a third addressed a focused clinical question, and only half provided an estimate of the magnitude of potential benefits [4].

Good review methods are important to give the reader an unbiased view of the state of current knowledge. Two problems occur in using research to answer specific questions. First, there is the problem of bias, either in our choice of which research to use, or within the research itself. So to minimise this, our review methods should attempt to identify and use the research with least bias. The second problem is that much research is based on samples that are too small, so we are at risk of type II errors, that is, concluding that a treatment or factor has no effect when the sample was too small to reliably rule out an important effect. The statistical methods of meta-analysis aim to combine studies to provide greater statistical power to answer a specific question. The problem with a non-systematic review is the potential for bias in answering questions, that is, that we choose the studies we like the results of or happen to know about rather than the best quality research.

For a systematic review of a single question, the usual format is the same as for most research papers, that is, Introduction, Methods, Results, And Discussion (IMRAD – see Chapters 1–5). Table 12.1 shows the likely elements of these sections. Though the other types of review may not fit this simple IMRAD structure, it is still worth considering each of these in developing and writing the review, even if the final structure varies from this. However, a review needs to be easily readable and you may need to deviate from the IMRAD structure for the sake of readability, but make sure these elements are still present.

Table 12.1 Structure for reporting a systematic review

Section	Contents
Introduction	Sets out the problem, and the specific questions addressed in the review
Methods	Describes the search and appraisal processes
	Often describes the number of studies checked and found eligible
Results	Describes the quality and results of eligible studies
Discussion	Summarises findings and their limitations and the implications for practice and research

The reviewing process

The steps and objectives in producing a good review are listed in Table 12.2. This chapter will give a brief description of each, but there are also several good texts that provide more extensive descriptions of the processes involved [5–7].

Table 12.2 Steps in a systematic review

Step	Processes
Formulate researchable questions	Set out the answerable question(s)
Find studies	Databases and search terms
Appraising quality	Quality criteria used to select studies
Synthesis	Methods of interpreting and/or combining results

Formulating questions

It can be helpful to break a research question down into components. For questions about treatment, the usual format is to identify the **P**atient group, the **I**ntervention of interest, suitable **C**omparison, and appropriate **O**utcome measures (PICO). For example, **P** – in patients with a history of stroke or transient ischaemic attacks are **I** – statins effective compared with **C** – no cholesterol lowering treatment for preventing **O** – the risk of ischaemic stroke.

While this seems a little artificial, it is a good discipline for clarifying the exact question addressed. The structure is less applicable to non-treatment questions, but can be adapted so that for diagnostic questions the 'I' is an index test, for prognosis, the 'I' is an indicator (or more traditionally an exposure, giving PECO).

Finding the studies

A systematic review of a focused question should clearly set out the search methods used.

Ideally the description of search methods should be included in the final report and briefly state the databases searched and the terms used for searching. The databases used will depend on the topic. For most clinical topics Medline is clearly essential but others such as Embase or CINAHL might also be relevant.

To devise appropriate search terms, it is helpful to use the PICO elements of the question to guide the search. Usually the P and I are the key elements as we may be interested in several outcomes. So the general process is to think of synonyms (which we combine with OR) for the P and I elements and combine these (with AND). For each synonym consider both text words and MeSH terms.

To reduce the searching workload, a useful technique is a 'methodological filter' which aims to find the best study type for each research question. A good example of this can be found on the PubMed interface to MEDLINE: the Clinical Queries tool. This provides empirically derived filters for five types of questions: aetiology, diagnosis, therapy, prognosis, and clinical prediction guides. If you are interested in the detailed terms used and their justification see the Filter Table linked on the Clinical Queries page.

Assessing study quality

A crucial element of the review process is sifting the good from the poor research, and basing conclusions, where possible, on the better research. To do that requires knowing what is the best possible evidence for each type of question. The first element of quality is the overall study design: was it a trial or a cohort study or a collection of cases?

Table 12.3 shows a hierarchy of evidence for different types of research questions. But this hierarchy is just a first cut – a useful time saver so that if you find good quality high-level studies, you may not need to read all the other papers [8].

Using Table 12.3 as a guide can save considerable time by reducing the number of articles you need to carefully examine. But be aware that there are times when a single case report can be convincing evidence of a treatment effect [9].

Synthesise

It is rare for all studies to reach the same conclusion, so a means of resolution is needed. However, a simple majority vote is dangerous. It will give as much weight to a large well-performed study as a small weaker study. For example, in the first systematic review of streptokinase for treating myocardial infarction only 5 of the 24 individual trials were 'statistically significant', but this was because almost all the trials were small and underpowered to detect the benefit [10]. So ideally, you should undertake a meta-analysis to resolve apparent differences. But a minimal alternative would be to focus initially on the largest high-quality study first and then contrast other studies with this main study.

Table 12.3 Designation of levels of evidence according to type of research question

Level	Intervention	Diagnosis	Prognosis	Aetiology
I	Systematic review of level II studies	Systematic reviewof level II studies	Systematic review of level II studies	Systematic review of level II studies
II	Randomised controlled trial	Cross-sectional study among consecutive presenting patients	Inception cohort study	Prospective cohort study
III	One of the following: non-randomised experimental study (e.g. controlled pre- and post-test intervention study), comparative (observational) study with a concurrent control group (e.g. cohort study, case-control study)	One of the following: cross-sectional study among non-consecutive patients, diagnostic case-control study	One of the following: untreated control patients in a randomised controlled trial, retrospectively assembled cohort study	One of the following: retrospective cohort study case-control study (*Note*: These are the most common study types for aetiology, but see level III for intervention studies for other options)
IV	Case series	Case series	Case series, or a cohort study of patients at different stages of disease	A cross-sectional study

However, even the largest study is sometimes insufficient. For example, in a systematic review of self-monitoring of anticoagulation [11], no single study showed a significant mortality benefit, but when combined the results were significant. Figure 12.1 shows the typical 'forest plot' of a meta-analysis, where we can see the confidence intervals of the individual trials cross the centre line (and hence are not statistically significant) but that the 'diamond' giving the pooled results doesn't include the odds ratio of 1, and hence is significant. Even if results are not pooled, such a graphical illustration of individual trial results is very helpful to readers.

Review:	Self-management for oral anticoagulation				
Comparison:	04 Death				
Outcome:	05 All trials				

Study or sub-category	Self-management n/N	Control n/N	OR (fixed) 95% CI	Weight (%)	OR (fixed) 95% CI
White (1989)	0/26	0/24			Not estimable
Sawicki (1999)	1/83	1/82		1.78	0.99 [0.06, 16.06]
Beyth (2000)	21/163	26/162		40.66	0.77 [0.42, 1.44]
Katz	0/101	0/100			Not estimable
Kortke (2001)	0/305	0/295			Not estimable
Sidhu (2001)	0/34	4/48		6.61	0.14 [0.01, 2.75]
Fitzmaurice (2002)	0/23	1/26		2.47	0.36 [0.01, 9.32]
Gardiner (2004)	1/29	0/24		0.93	2.58 [0.10, 66.24]
Sunderji (2004)	0/69	0/70			Not estimable
Fitzmaurice (2005)	5/337	11/280		21.18	0.37 [0.13, 1.07]
Menendez-Jandula (2005)	6/368	15/369		26.37	0.39 [0.15, 1.02]
Voller (2005)	0/101	0/101			Not estimable
Total (95% CI)	**1639**	**1581**		**100.00**	**0.56 [0.36, 0.86]**

Total events: 34 (self-management), 58 (control)
Test for hetero geneity: Chi^2 = 4.07, df = 6 (p = 0.67), I^2 = 0%
Test for overall effect: Z = 2.64 (p = 0.008)

0.1 0.2   0.5   1   2   5   10
Favours self-manage   Favours control

Figure 12.1 Meta-analytic 'forest plot' of the effects seen in trials of self-monitoring of INR (updated by Rafael Perera from Heneghan [11]).

Of course, numerical meta-analysis can only be undertaken for quantitative data but it is also possible to be systematic in combining qualitative data [12]. The main principle is to avoid basing conclusions on your prior preferences, but instead to base statements on the best quality evidence.

Conclusions

In conclusion, the review process might be summarised as follows: empty your mind of fixed opinions, take a methodical and critical approach to research literature, then describe what you found in an engaging manner.

References

1 Booth, WC, Colomb GG, Williams JM. *The craft of research*, 2nd edn. 2003 Series: Chicago Guides to Writing, Editing, and Publishing, Chicago: The University of Chicago Press, 2003.
2 McGee S, Abernethy 3rd WB, Simel DL. The rational clinical examination. Is this patient hypovolemic? *JAMA* 1999;**281**:1022–9.
3 Sackett DL. The rational clinical examination. A primer on the precision and accuracy of the clinical examination. *JAMA* 1992;**267**:2638–44.
4 McAlister FA, Clark HD, van Walraven C, Straus SE, Lawson FM, Moher D, Mulrow CD. The medical review article revisited: has the science improved? *Ann Intern Med* 1999;**131**:947–51.
5 Glasziou P, Irwig P, Bain C, Colditz G. *Systematic reviews in health care: a practical guide*. Cambridge: Cambridge University Press, 2001.
6 Khan KS, Kunz R, Kleijnen J, Antes G. *Systematic reviews to support evidence-based medicine. How to review and apply findings of health care research*. London: RSM Press, 2003.
7 Mulrow C, Cook D, eds. *Systematic reviews: synthesis of best evidence for health care decisions*. Philadelphia: American College of Physicians, 1998.
8 Glasziou PP, Vandenbroucke J, Chalmers I. Assessing the quality of research. *BMJ* 2004;**328**:39–41.
9 Glasziou P, Chalmers I, Rawlins M, McCulloch P. When are randomised trials unnecessary? Picking signal from noise. *BMJ* 2007;**334**:349–51.
10 Stampfer MJ, Goldhaber SZ, Yusuf S, Peto R, Hennekens CH. Effect of intravenous streptokinase on acute myocardial infarction: pooled results from randomized trials. *New Engl J Med* 1982;**307**:1180–2.
11 Heneghan C, Alonso-Coello P, Garcia-Alamino J, Perera R, Meats E, Glasziou P. Self-monitoring of oral anticoagulation: a systematic review and meta-analysis. *Lancet* 2006;**367**:404–11.
12 Lucas PJ, Baird J, Arai L, Law C, Roberts HM. Worked examples of alternative methods for the synthesis of qualitative and quantitative research in systematic reviews. *BMC Med Res Methodol* 2007;**7**:4.

Chapter 13 **The role of the editor**

Jennifer M. Hunter

Editors are simple souls: they have to be to survive the heavy workload of a never-ending round of new manuscripts, revised manuscripts, Letters to the Editor, ethical issues and complaints, to name but a few. But they must also be well-organised individuals, with significant administrative skills, a degree of impetuosity, and a huge work ethic. They must try to maintain, at all times, clarity of thought and a clear vision. They also very much need a sense of humour.

Authors must appreciate that, whatever they submit to the Editor-in-Chief (EIC) of a scientific journal, however long or short, it is just a small moment in that editor's life. More importantly, that editor is so busy that he or she wants every new arrival in his mailbox (electronic or hard copy) to be problem free. Thus he approves Guidelines to Authors to be published in each issue of the journal, for authors to follow meticulously, paying significant attention to detail.

The EIC is the pivotal link between the author and the expert assessor: they will at all times attempt to ensure that fair play is maintained, and that the author's voice is heard. To encourage such behaviour, authors should in every way possible provide the EIC with exactly what is required of them. (Always try to humour an editor – it pays dividends in profusion.) It is wise to ask a senior colleague with significant publishing experience to read over a manuscript before it is submitted to an editor. None of us, however experienced, fails to benefit from this approach.

In this short chapter, I will cover the commonplace aspects of an editor's role: to them alone will the real anguish, frustrations and anxieties of the job be known [1].

New manuscripts

Every morning begins in an active Editorial Office by considering newly submitted manuscripts. With the aid of expert secretarial support, each new manuscript must be checked in detail. Has it been submitted correctly? Are the subsections correctly named (Summary, Introduction, Methods, Results, Discussion, etc.)? Are the tables and figures legible, and presented if necessary in the correct electronic format? Are the figures and tables actually mentioned in the text (a common omission), and are they labelled correctly? Often the number of tables and figures provided by an author does not correspond to the number mentioned in the text. Is the word count within the maximum permitted by the journal, and are the Declarations of Interest and completed Copyright forms provided? Have all the authors signed the Conflict of Interest form and submission letter, if appropriate? Indeed, do all the authors know that they have contributed to this paper?

On receipt of a new manuscript which meets all the necessary submission criteria, an EIC will allocate the manuscript to one of their editorial team who has some knowledge of the subject under discussion. Alternatively, they will take responsibility for the manuscript themselves. The responsible editor will invite at least two and probably three expert assessors to comment on it. (Even numbers of assessors produce the problem for editors of split decisions; if an odd number of assessors is used, then a majority recommendation is likely.)

Immediate rejection

Occasionally, it is immediately obvious to an EIC that the manuscript has been submitted inappropriately: the topic would be more suitably considered by another speciality journal, or the standard of the science or the use of English is well below the minimum required by that journal. Only at the most 5% of new manuscripts fall into this category. In such an instance, the EIC will not hesitate to take an immediate decision, which is usually 'Reject'. However, a thoughtful editor will often accompany this decision by detailed advice to the author on how the manuscript could be improved significantly.

Revised manuscripts

As the number of revisions of a manuscript increases so does the detailed contribution of the editor to it. Once you have been asked by an editor to submit a revision of your manuscript, always take on the task eagerly and with delight – your foot is through the door! Do not be discouraged if the demands seem extensive and excessive; consider each of them in detail, and act on at least some of them. Ultimately, you will reply to the editor, detailing systematically how you have responded to each of the assessors' comments. The editor will not expect you to do exactly what each assessor suggests – not every comment or criticism can possibly be completely apt – but you must be prepared to argue your point in each instance. At this stage, the editor acts as a 'go between': he will hear the author's voice as much as the assessor's. At all times, try to be courteous in your response, whatever the frustrations you experience. By approaching this exercise in a balanced, professional manner, you will make greater progress (Box 13.1).

Box 13.1 How to please an editor

- Adhere strictly to the Guidelines for Authors throughout the text.
- Do exactly what the Guidelines dictate: no more, no less. Make the editor's life easier.
- Avoid basic errors such as incorrect numbering of figures or tables; forgetting to attach figures and using the wrong reference format.
- If invited to submit a revision, attend to every detail raised by the editor and assessors in a structured, unemotional manner.
- Contact the Editorial Office if you are concerned that your manuscript is not being dealt with efficiently.
- Communicate courteously and correctly with the Editorial Office, arguing your case coherently and professionally.
- Never submit a manuscript to more than one journal simultaneously: editors find out, and they loathe the practice.
- Make sure that all the authors have read and contributed to the manuscript. Would they be willing to stand up in public to defend their work?

Never submit a manuscript labelled 'revised version' when it is almost unchanged from the first draft. Few things irritate an editor more than an author asking for a revised version to be considered when it is in essence the same as the first version. It does happen. How could an author possibly think that an editor would be so foolish as not to notice?

Problem manuscripts

Some authors respond rapidly to the request for a revision of a manuscript; others do not reply for many months. It is the EIC's role to check when replies from assessors or authors are not received. Have they gone missing in the post or on the website? Has the author or assessor changed their address or email address (a common problem with trainee doctors in particular)? Always help an Editorial Office to keep fully up to date with all your contact details. Every EIC has, amongst the hundreds of manuscripts received each year, a very few that are almost 'jinxed': where, for instance, all the assessors take a very long time to reply, and then provide an inane or inadequate critique. It is the editor's responsibility to provide the authors in every instance with a critical appraisal of their paper: one which will help to improve the quality of the manuscript, or possibly the research in question. An editor may therefore have on occasion to ask for a rapid yet thorough appraisal of a manuscript, for which he has not yet obtained a satisfactory report. This is one example of the role of an Editorial Board to a scientific editor: it should be possible for an editor to ask a Board member to produce such a report proficiently in these circumstances.

Thus an Editorial Office will, with the help of modern electronic manuscript tracking systems, be able very regularly to check that every manuscript under active review by their journal is being handled expeditiously. They must set time aside at least once a month to check that no manuscript has been delayed unacceptably when undergoing peer review. An EIC owes that to an author, if nothing else. Authors should, however, never hesitate to contact an Editorial Office if they have had no contact about their manuscript for several weeks (Box 13.1). Errors do happen even in the most efficiently run Editorial Office.

Rejected manuscripts

Most speciality journals have a rejection rate of over 60%. Thus a significant number of manuscripts will be rejected, not because they make no scientific contribution, but because they are not in the top 40% of submissions scientifically. Rejection is a disappointment to any author: editors know that for they have usually experienced it themselves. Authors are often angry and frustrated when their manuscript is rejected and retort vociferously to the editor. The more senior the author, the greater is the aggression. Try not to be too personal or rude in your response in such circumstances. You have the right of reply, but it will be considered more fully if it is balanced and logical. Often another assessor (who is unaware that your manuscript has already been rejected) will be asked to review it. In general, however, it is unusual for such a decision to be completely overturned on appeal.

Editorials, reviews and correspondence

An EIC must ensure that for each issue at least one editorial and scientific review are published. These contributions come from experts who can usually write well and with ease. They are not therefore difficult to edit. But they can be difficult to obtain, for international authorities are exceptionally busy, and used to missing publishing deadlines. An EIC must approach such experts with care and respect, knowing that their journal and its impact factor, will very possibly be improved by such a contribution. An EIC will therefore have a list of editorials and reviews to hand, all at various stages of development. The Editorial Board of a journal are expected regularly to support the EIC in this respect, by producing such manuscripts themselves, and by inviting contributions of a high standard.

Books are also submitted very regularly by publishers to an Editorial Office for review. This is not a particularly arduous task for an EIC, although again, experts who agree to review books must often be cajoled into returning their report expeditiously. An EIC wants to have new books reviewed rapidly in their journal, and to beat their competitors into publishing them.

Letters to the Editor in contrast, flow in, day after day, hour upon hour, without any invitation. The standard of writing is often poor, even when a valid point or contribution is being made. The EIC, or one of his editorial team, takes responsibility for editing this constant stream, which is a significant part of the day-to-day running of a scientific journal. Letters are now often submitted electronically to a journal website. This approach has the advantage of more rapid handling and turnover, which is particularly important when comments are being made about a prospective scientific study, or when an equipment fault or adverse drug reaction is reported. The editor can then speed up the submission to publication time. An electronic website also encourages more readers to comment, which is important to any editor [2]. It has the disadvantage, however, of encouraging submissions to which insufficient attention to detail has been given. It is worth an author making significant effort if they wish to get their letter into print. The selection of letters from the website for publication in print will be decided not only by the message contained therein but also by the ease of understanding it.

Occasionally, an editor will ask for an expert opinion on a Letter to the Editor, especially when it is not written about a recently published article in a journal. Do not be surprised therefore to receive a full scientific assessment of your correspondence.

Handling correspondence is a significant burden to any editor: it never goes away. But it must be done well for readers enjoy a vibrant correspondence section in any journal. It is often the most commonly read part of an issue.

Assembling an issue

One of the more creative and hence enjoyable tasks for an EIC is to put together the monthly contents of their journal. They must encourage and cajole their editorial team into editing manuscripts accurately, yet efficiently, so that the Acceptance to Publication intervals are kept as short as possible. In this respect too, editors are competing with other scientific journals in their field: if authors know that a journal has a good reputation for handling manuscripts efficiently, they are more likely to submit papers to it. Hence that journal will receive higher-quality articles for consideration and publication, which will hopefully improve its impact factor. Publication ahead of print on the journal's website has shortened the Acceptance to Publication time significantly for many journals [3]. In addition, by a process known as *Open Access*, many journals now invite authors to pay for the full text of their article to be available on the journal website as soon as it is accepted for publication. Larger journals, such as the *BMJ*, do not even charge a fee for this facility [3].

Impact factor

Every editor must believe in the principle of the impact factor, and at all times aim to improve it for their journal, whatever its limitations [4]. No better measure of a journal's scientific content is available and every Editorial Board works to improve it for their journal. Thus, despite their busy daily routine, an EIC must set aside time for detailed consideration with their Editorial Team and Board of how the contents of their journal can be improved. Will, for instance, removing Short Reports, which are rarely cited, or Case Reports, improve their journal's impact factor [5]? If so, and it is possible for editors to study the effect of such changes on their journal's impact factor, then changes must be effected to a journal's content, and rapidly. It is difficult for an EIC not to become oppressed by adverse changes in their journal's impact factor: their attitude to it must in many ways be schizoid. They must be fiercely keen to improve it, but recognise its statistical limitations and quirks.

Appearance of a scientific journal

Editors realise that 'beauty is in the eye of the beholder'. Any journal, whether it be scientific, political or a leisure magazine, must be attractive to the eye. The reader must enjoy handling it and know their way around it. Yet a reader appreciates small, subtle, but regular changes which catch their attention. They do not want the image of any journal to be the same year on year. Thus the EIC must consider with his editorial team, board and publisher, regular changes to the appearance of the journal and its layout. These are items which the scientific publisher can often advise upon, and can detail the limitations under which the editor must work in this respect.

Advertisements in scientific journals, which are often an important source of regular income, must also be checked by the EIC with the publisher – to avoid embarrassment over inaccuracies, outrageous claims or factual errors. Each scientific journal has its own rules, of which the publisher must be fully aware, as to where it is acceptable to place advertisements in an issue. For instance, few EICs will allow an advertisement to break up the text of a research paper, but some will allow one between sections for example between the Editorials and Scientific Reviews.

Team play

An EIC is the leader of a team of highly intelligent editors, who have busy professional lives stretching far beyond the journal. An EIC must ensure that no editor or assessor is over-burdened, or else that member of the team will perform their journal work less well [6]. The EIC must also ensure that the relationship between the editorial and publishing staff is harmonious, and effective and efficient, and must detect disquiet early so that it can be rapidly corrected. Despite the many heavy pressures of their office, an EIC must, as with any senior administrator, ensure at all times that their team is content. They must meet regularly to discuss problems, in circumstances where they cannot be easily disturbed.

Transparency

An EIC must also ensure, in this present climate, that the daily functioning of their journal is completely transparent [7]. An author or reader should be able to access the journal's website, which is usually written with the publisher, to obtain full details of the journal's policies on such issues as: Conflicts of Interest of authors, assessors and editors; the assessment process; appointment and payment of the Editorial team; and appointment of the Editorial board. It is ultimately the EIC's responsibility to ensure that all these aspects of a journal's image are up to date and of the required standard.

Complaints

Authors must always sense that an Editorial Office has 'an open door' policy, that it is easy to contact and communicate with. An EIC should lead this office by example, rapidly and reliably answering all queries that are received each day, and they do pour in, by telephone, email (increasingly), facsimile and post. The image of any journal is not enhanced if the author receives no response to their enquiry; the author's voice must always be heard.

Complaints are extremely time-consuming for an EIC. They must be investigated in detail and an appropriate response made, if necessary by a published apology such as an Erratum notice in the journal. Errors in a busy Editorial Office are inevitable, and the EIC must take full responsibility for them even if they have been made by one of their team. An EIC must track down the cause of the error and correct it as rapidly as possible. They can be made by the publisher, the author or the editorial team.

In contrast, an EIC must at all times be wary of the author who is trying to fool or confuse any of the editorial team and without doubt such authors, often very intelligent ones, exist. Their motive may be mischievous or personal, competitive or exhibitionist: an EIC must be able to deal with a huge range of personalities. Ideally, an EIC will have a broad albeit at times shallow knowledge of their speciality. An expert in a small even if important subspeciality is not as easily able to deal with the breadth of scientific and ethical challenges presented to them.

Ethical issues

At any time, an EIC will be dealing with several examples of poor conduct by authors, or indeed by assessors or editors. These must be dealt with strictly and to the highest standards. The Committee of Publication Ethics (COPE) [8] publish detailed guidelines to help editors to handle such issues (http://www.publicationethics.org.uk).

Confirming that the correct details have been established in issues of plagiarism, dual or redundant publication, or fraudulent data (misconduct) are very time-consuming for an EIC, but must at all times be dealt with propitiously [9]. Liaison is often necessary with editors of other scientific journals who perhaps have published the article first (and whose first language may not be English). International handling of confidential information requires patient attention to detail, and the highest of moral standards.

Authors also have the right to know that their manuscript is undergoing such investigation. They must be kept fully informed of the process of any EIC's investigation, and be given the right of reply. EICs have no legal authority; they can only request clarification and take such appropriate action as they consider reasonable to maintain the highest ethical standards of publishing for their journal [10]. This often involves publishing a formal apology in a clear position such as at the end of the editorials in their journal. It also often requires contacting the employer of the offender such as the Dean of their medical school to keep them fully informed of the problem [7].

Confidentiality

All communications received by an EIC must be considered confidential, whatever their nature. An EIC owes it to an author not only to treat their work with such respect but to ensure that all his editorial team, of whatever grade, appreciate this too.

Conclusions

Being an EIC of a scientific journal is a highly privileged albeit onerous role. One EIC has compared it to having a demanding mistress [1]! EICs spend all their professional hours in the public, indeed international eye. They must at all times strive to maintain the highest possible scientific and ethical standards for their journal. Inevitably, there will be times when they fail, but hopefully these will be few in number.

References

1 Harmer M. A moment to reflect. *Anaesthesia* 2003;**88**:1159–61.
2 Hunter JM. A fond farewell. *Br J Anaesth* 2005;**94**:145–6.
3 Groves T. Why submit your research to the *BMJ*? *BMJ* 2007;**334**:4–5.
4 Smith G. Impact factors in anaesthesia journals. *Br J Anaesth* 1996;**76**:753–4.
5 Hunter JM. The latest changes ... no more shorts. *Br J Anaesth* 2004;**92**:7.
6 Smith G. Personal reflections. *Br J Anaesth* 1997;**79**:1–2.
7 Todd MM. The best years of my life. *Anesthesiology* 2007;**106**:1–2.
8 Committee on Publication Ethics (1999 and 2003). *Guidelines on good publication practice*. The COPE Report, London, BMJ Publishing Group.
9 Hunter JM. Plagiarism – does the punishment fit the crime? *Vet Anaesth Analg* 2006;**33**:139–42.
10 Hunter JM. Ethics in publishing: are we practising to the highest possible standards? *Br J Anaesth* 2000;**85**:341–3.

Chapter 14 **The role of the manuscript assessor**

Domhnall MacAuley

Introduction

Reviewing a paper. How can you help the editor, help the author, and get the most out of the experience? This chapter will look at the process of assessment: how your review can be of most value to the editor when he or she makes a decision about acceptance, rejection, or revision. If the decision is to reject, it will also help the author improve their manuscript for resubmission or future submission to another journal.

Every manuscript is important. For the author, it is the final stage in the long and increasingly complex process of undertaking a research project. It is not just the communication of findings but also of individual career enhancement and institutional esteem. After endless hours of work – drafting and redrafting, negotiating with coauthors, checking tables and graphs, collating signatures, and massaging egos – the paper is finally completed and dispatched. And you, the reviewer, are contacted shortly afterwards, with a polite note from the editor asking if you would be willing to give your opinion.

Remember, you were once that author. If you have been asked to review a paper, you are almost certainly involved in a research career and have published a number of papers. You will remember how you sent off your first paper – nervous, anxious, and excited – and awaited the response and reviewer's opinion. You read every detail of the review, studying every word of the critique, analysing, and reanalysing their meaning. You grumbled if the reviewer did not appear to understand your work, were thrilled at words of encouragement, were irritated if they did not seem up to date with the latest literature, and argued with their interpretation of the findings. So, be kind. It is a privilege to be asked to give an opinion on someone else's work, but with this invitation is a responsibility to do it well. The author may be a senior and experienced academic but many papers are submitted by inexperienced authors setting out on their career. This may be the author's first tentative step into the world of academia. Be helpful. Be the reviewer that you would have liked to review your first paper, and don't try to show how good you are. Be thorough and detailed. Above all, be fair and honest.

The role of reviewer gives little reward. Academic publishing is based on the generosity and altruism of researchers and requires a lot of work with little return. Most journals do not pay for reviews, and only recently has reviewing been recognised as a measure of academic esteem by universities. Good reviewing requires idealism and is a thankless task that takes time and effort to do well [1]. The primary reward is in the contribution the reviewer makes to the research community. It takes time, and reviewers, on average, spend 2–4 h and review for 3.6 journals [2]. When reviewers decline, it is usually because of lack of time, or that the paper is not relevant to their area of interest or expertise [3].

Specialist versus generalist journals

Specialist and general journals may have different needs and expectations. In a specialist journal, the editor usually asks two or more reviewers to assess a paper. The editor's knowledge is unlikely to span the entire breadth of the journal's range, so they need an expert opinion. The final decision on how to deal with the paper will be made by the editor alone, but having two or more opinions gives editors more confidence in their decision.

In large general journals, although an editor may not be expert in a particular field, there is likely to be a larger editorial faculty, with the paper passing through more than one editorial committee and seen by a number of assessors before subsequent acceptance or rejection. The reviewer's opinion carries considerable weight in the final decision in each case, but this opinion is only one part of the decision process and may be interpreted differently in different journals. Sometimes, although it is unusual, an editor may accept a paper of which the reviewer is unsupportive or reject a paper that the reviewer thinks should be published. In general, however, the reviewer does have considerable influence on the editorial decision.

The process

Electronic publishing has revolutionised paper handling, and an invitation to review often comes by email. You retrieve the abstract by a website or portal which then allows you to decide if you know enough about the topic to undertake the review. The decision to review or not can be difficult. If you are not an expert in the field or are certain that you cannot complete the review in time, do let the editor know by return. If you have doubts about your time availability, respond immediately and decline – few people find that their days become less cluttered. If you can do it, however, please do. You will be asked to give your opinion by a particular date, usually 3–4 weeks from receipt. When you reply you will receive an electronic response, often instantaneous, thanking you and giving you access to the full paper. You may need Adobe Acrobat to read the paper; if you do not have the appropriate software, the journal will usually give you guidance on how to download it. You may also have access to an electronic response form to submit your review. Alternatively, you may write your review on a word processor and attach or upload the file.

If you cannot complete the review in the time indicated, do let the editorial assistant and editor know as soon as possible. It is much better to know that a reviewer cannot help than for nobody to know what is happening. Yes, we have all been guilty – a paper for review sitting at the bottom of a pile of work, never quite making it to the top. Do try to complete it on time, otherwise the editorial assistant will have to chase you and it seems that the only way to get reviewers to produce on time is to remind them [4].

Occasionally, you will be asked to review a paper where you know little about the topic. Major journals have large electronic databases that can be searched with keywords identified from information that you, as a previous author or potential reviewer, have submitted yourself. Alternatively, the editor may have found your name on a database or identified you as an author on a paper on this or a related topic. Electronic databases, for example, often provide the email address of the corresponding author. This may not always be the best method to identify potential reviewers. Young ambitious academics tend to move jobs and universities fairly regularly, and the email address may be obsolete; interests change, so a paper published 3 years ago may reflect work carried out 3 or more years previously; or the corresponding author may not always be the overall expert behind the work. Mistakes happen, so be patient with editors, and do let us know as soon as possible if we have made an error!

On the other hand, an editor may have had difficulty identifying a reviewer with expertise in a particular specialist field and you may have been asked because you have a related interest. If, in these circumstances, you can write a review, please do. It might be a bit more difficult because you might have to read around the topic, but do give it some thought. Some papers appear jinxed, in that every potential reviewer approached declines and the editor is left with a list of refusals from reviewers and an increasingly anxious author who has waited a long time for an opinion.

Journals often invite authors to suggest potential reviewers. This may seem open to potential problems. But, it appears to be less flawed than one might anticipate. There is evidence that author and editor suggested reviewers do not differ in the actual quality of their reviews. But, author suggested reviewers were more favourable in their recommendations for acceptance. So, editors can be confident in the assessment of the paper, but would be best advised to make their own judgement on acceptance [5].

And, please forgive the poor editor who mistakenly invites you to review a paper you have submitted yourself. In searching topic codes, they identify the perfect reviewer, someone who has written extensively on the subject and who would clearly be the ideal assessor, but forget to scan the author list. It happens.

The best and the worst reviews

The perfect review does not exist. Neither of course, does the perfect manuscript. But, the best review is one that informs both the editor and the author of the limitations and possible improvements to a piece of work.

The editor, primarily, needs to know if it is suitable for publication and how it can be improved. If the work has fatal flaws, usually in relation to the method, this makes the decision to reject much easier. If the paper could be acceptable with modification, the editor needs to know if this is possible. Minor problems can be corrected easily.

The best reviewer reads around the topic. With such easy access to electronic databases at hospitals, at universities, and on home computers, an editor expects the assessor to do a brief search of the literature to be able to comment on the originality of the work.

No strict guidelines exist on the structure of a review, but a general consensus seems to have evolved that divides the review into three parts. The first part is usually a general comment on the paper – its originality, importance, and validity. The second part deals with major problems, and the third part lists minor problems. This structure can be used in any review and is a delight to the editor and author.

A helpful review begins with a short summary that places the paper in context and essentially answers the twin questions: is it new and is it true? This means giving an opinion on the originality of a piece of work; if the findings have been reported previously and, how much this particular manuscript adds to the current literature. The reviewer should indicate if, in the context of their specialist knowledge, the subject matter or research question is of sufficient importance and novelty that it merits publication. Asking if it is true, is really a question about the method. It means deciding if the method used in the research is sound. This requires some knowledge of basic epidemiological principles but doesn't usually require statistical expertise. Most journals seek a further statistician's opinion. The assessor should also know enough about the journal to know whether the style and content fits within the remit or range of interest of the journal.

Example
Summary

> This is an interesting and well-written paper on peer review. The authors have identified an important research question and have addressed it in an organised and well-structured paper. It is a useful new contribution to the literature because it demonstrates that peer review does help improve the quality of a paper, and there is very little high-quality research on this topic. The paper is well written and fits with the style of the *Journal of Medical Writing*. I have some major concerns about the sampling method and some minor concerns about the accuracy of writing.

The second section of the review may identify major criticisms of the paper. It will address the relevance and appropriateness of the introduction, problems identified in the methods, the accuracy of the results, the interpretation of these results in the discussion, and the objectivity and validity of the conclusion. Each problem should be referenced to the text of the paper by using the page number, paragraph number, and line number if possible. Direct quotations included in the review should be in parentheses. This allows both the editor and the author to look to the text and locate the problem immediately. Major criticisms should be highlighted as fatal flaws that would prevent publication of the paper.

Example
Major criticisms

> Page 2, paragraph 2, line 3. The authors describe their sampling method. Allocation by day of arrival of a manuscript is not an acceptable method of randomisation in a randomised controlled trial.
> Page 2, paragraph 2, line 7. The authors do not identify the inclusion and exclusion criteria.

The third section lists minor criticisms, and it may include advice on possible improvements to the introduction, suggestions for additional references, and comments on the context of the paper and errors in spelling and grammar.

Example
Minor criticisms

> Page 1, paragraph 3, line 2. The introduction covers the literature appropriately, although the authors may like to look at two other papers on randomised controlled trials (Godlee *et al.* and van Royen *et al.*).
>
> Page 1, paragraph 3, line 4. Misspelling of the word trial – spelt 'trail'.

Case reports are treated differently. Some journals publish case reports regularly and others only in special circumstances. The *BMJ*, for example, does not publish case reports unless they are submitted as a 'lesson of the week'. The decision to publish a case report usually pivots on its originality. The author may believe that theirs is an original observation but reviewers should check the literature. Similar cases may have been reported in a different field, language, or country and have not been reported previously in this specialty or geographical location. Different editors use different criteria, and the role of the reviewer is to provide enough information to allow the editor to make a decision.

Improving the quality

The peer review process has evolved as a method of objective selection on scientific merit. It is, however, at best, an inexact science, and there is poor evidence that peer review gives a better decision in the end. Indeed, a recent systematic review from the international Cochrane Collaboration (http://www.nelh.nhs.uk) concluded that little hard evidence showed that peer review improved the quality of published biomedical research [6]. It is also difficult to measure the quality of peer review, with little agreement on measures of quality [7].

A number of randomised controlled trials have been conducted on blinding or open peer review [8,9]. Fiona Godlee, one of the key researchers in the field, puts the case that open review is superior ethically to anonymous reviews and that open review increases the accountability of the reviewers, with less scope for biased or unjustified judgements or misappropriation of data under the cloak of anonymity. With blinded review, complete blinding is difficult and 23–42% of reviewers not told the identity of authors were able to identify them [10]. Papers nearly always include some reference to the location or special nature of the population being examined. Most researchers know the other researchers in a specialist field and can often identify their work.

In the interests of honesty and transparency, journals may opt for open peer review. In this system, both the author and the reviewer know each other's identity. Some argue that reviewers may be less likely to give an incisive and critical review, but it also protects the author from the unscrupulous reviewer. Although relatively few journals have adopted this system at present, it is likely to become more common in response to increasing pressure to open up the entire process of peer review.

Open review does have possible disadvantages. It may increase the number of reviewers who decline to review, the likelihood that reviewers will recommend acceptance, and the time taken to produce a report. It is also possible that junior reviewers would be less likely to give an honest criticism of work by senior colleagues. Threats – overt or covert – and bullying by more senior academics are possible. In order to protect reviewers, when the *BMJ* introduced its open peer review [11], it also introduced a system of anonymous notification of intimidation of reviewers. They termed this the yellow card system, because of its similarity to the drug adverse reaction notification system in the United Kingdom. The *BMJ* has received only a few yellow cards since introducing open review. With open review, the author may try to take their complaint directly to the reviewer, rather than going through the editorial process. This, of course, is inappropriate. In such cases, the reviewer should not respond directly but should contact the editor directly. This allows both parties to take a step back from any confrontation and passes responsibility to the editor to settle any differences.

Bias – conscious or subconscious – is always a possibility. A reviewer may be tempted to favour a former collaborator's work or may have a tendency to be more critical of the work of a competitor. But, when an author reads a review and feels their paper has been dealt with harshly, it may not be bias but simply that the reviewer may, because of their specialist knowledge, know more about the potential pitfalls and mistakes involved in research in a particular area.

Editors are also very interested in looking at methods to improve the quality of peer review. Training peer reviewers through workshops, training programmes, or direct feedback may all have something to offer. However, direct feedback appears to be ineffective and indeed, may have a negative effect [12]. When we look at the outcomes of training initiatives, the results may not be what we might have expected. Training packages have only a minor impact on the quality of reviews of manuscripts. When comparing self-taught training with face-to-face training, the self-taught package appeared, statistically, to be slightly more effective but was not considered editorially significant and the effects were short lasting [13].

If you would like to find out more about improving the quality of your peer review, you may like to look at guidance on the website of the World Association of Medical Editors (http://www.wame.org/syllabus.htm#reviewers

and http://www.wame.org/wamestmt.htm). You might be interested in attending a training programme in peer review [14]. Or, if you are interested in what is happening in research into peer review you may wish to look at http://bmjresearch.com/

Dealing with an appeal

There is a increasing tendency for authors to appeal an editor's decision. This creates a dilemma. Everyone makes mistakes, and editors, perhaps more than most, are aware of the weaknesses of the peer review process and acutely aware that the system can fail. If an editor has any doubt that a paper may have been rejected unfairly, they will usually re-examine the decision. That process may include asking for a further review. In such cases, the editor will usually send all the correspondence, together with the previous review(s), to the new assessor and will ask for a further opinion. The assessor should go through exactly the same process of assessing the paper on its merits. The final decision will be with the editor, but as the reviewer, you are the consultant advisor, whose advice helps that decision.

Referee, reviewer, or assessor

The deliberate use of the term assessor or reviewer in this chapter is an attempt to move away from the term referee. Sometimes assessors find the task difficult and are uncomfortable making decisions about the work of their peers. It helps to remember, however, that the final decision is with the editor, and it is their responsibility. The use of the term referee can be misleading, because it is the editor who must make the decision. Your role, as reviewer, is to give an honest assessment of the value of a piece of work in the context of your knowledge, experience, and your brief review of the relevant literature.

Improving the quality of the review

Research suggests that the best peer reviewers are aged under 40 years, trained in epidemiology or statistics, and live in North America [15]. The quality of a review depends greatly on how much time and effort the reviewer is prepared to invest.

Do authors care? It is difficult to know, but one study of 897 corresponding authors of the *Annals of Emergency Medicine*, with a 64% response rate, showed modest satisfaction with peer review [16]. Those authors whose papers were accepted were most satisfied with peer review, and authors of rejected manuscripts were dissatisfied both with the time taken to decision and the communication from the editor. Authors were happy if their paper was accepted irrespective of review quality.

Conflict of interest

Reviewers do have an ethical responsibility. Assessors are chosen because of their interest in the particular field, so you may find yourself appraising the work of your former colleagues or your competitors. If this creates a conflict of interest, do let the editor know. The peer review process is based entirely on trust. It depends on your integrity and, just as you would expect an honest and true assessment of your work, so do your colleagues – even if they are your competitors. Authors sometimes submit their manuscripts with a request that the editor not use certain reviewers, who they feel may not give a fair assessment. Although we expect assessors to have the utmost integrity, most editors would consider such a request to be reasonable.

You also have a responsibility to maintain the integrity of the peer review system, however, and, if you think an author could possibly have any concern about your independence, do contact the editor. On the other hand, sometimes you may be the only person qualified to review a paper. Disclosure is the best protection against an accusation of conflict of interest. If you inform the editor and try to give an honest appraisal of the paper, you have done everything that you can do. The editor can then disclose to the author, if necessary, that you highlighted a potential conflict of interest.

You also have a responsibility for intellectual integrity; you must not use other people's ideas. It does happen – and can happen even subconsciously – so it is important to be on your guard.

The website of the World Association of Medical Editors (http://www.wame.org) is a very useful resource and provides extensive guidance on conflict of interest on their Topic list. It also includes a discussion on a case submitted anonymously by an editor and discussed at the Fourth International Congress on Peer Review in Barcelona in September 2001. The case, relating to a reviewer's financial interest, was presented to the audience by Michael Callaham of the WAME Ethics Committee and was discussed by an expert panel, consisting of Richard Smith (*BMJ*), Richard Horton (*Lancet*), and Frank Davidoff (*Annals of Internal Medicine*).

Research misconduct

You may, at times, as an assessor, have doubts about a paper. It may be that you doubt the figures, the tables, the complete reporting of results, manipulation of sampling, etc. If you suspect research misconduct, it is important that you bring your doubts to the attention of the editor. You could be wrong, however, so this must be done in a subtle and sensitive manner.

The editor has a number of options in such cases, but the most likely is that he or she will ask the author to supply the protocol, original data, information on sampling arrangements, a copy of the ethical approval, etc. This may uncover a mistake, a misreport, an error of judgement, or a deliberate attempt to mislead. As a reviewer, it is important not to make a judgement or accusation without serious consideration and a degree of certainty. If there is a problem or doubt, the editor may ask the Committee on Publication Ethics (COPE) to consider the case [17].

If you are concerned about duplicate or 'salami' publication, it is helpful if you send copies of other relevant papers so the editor can identify the degree of overlap. Academic departments are under huge pressure to publish as many papers as possible, and there may be the temptation to try to split a piece of work into multiple manuscripts to maximise the number of publications and increase the number of papers on a curriculum vitae. In the current academic climate, such salami publishing is understandable but inappropriate. It clutters up the literature and makes it difficult to identify the true message in any piece of work. Recent changes to the RAE in the UK may help.

Conclusion

It is an honour and a privilege to be asked to give a prepublication opinion on a colleague's work. The academic world depends on the altruism of researchers to ensure the continued existence of peer review. There is also a responsibility to do it well, however. Try to invest the time and effort into providing the type of review that you would like from an assessor if they had been asked to review your work.

References

1 Goldbeck-Wood S. What makes a good reviewer of manuscripts. *BMJ* 1998;**316**:86.

2 Yankaur A. Who are the peer reviewers and how much do they review. *JAMA* 1990;**263**:1338–40.

3 Tite L, Schroter S. Why do peer reviewers decline to review. A survey. *J Epidemiol Community Health* 2007;**61**:9–12.

4 Pitkin RM, Burmeister LF. Prodding tardy reviewers. *JAMA* 2002;**287**:2794–5.

5 Schroter S, Tite L, Hutchings, A, Black N. Differences in review quality and recommendations for publication between peer reviewers suggested by authors or by editors. *JAMA* 2006;**295**:314–7.

6 White C. Little evidence for effectiveness of scientific peer review. *BMJ* 2003;**326**:241.

7 Jefferson T, Wager E, Davidoff F. Measuring the quality of editorial peer review. *JAMA* 2002;**287**:2786–90.

8 Godlee F, Cale CR, Marlyn CN. Effect on the quality of peer review of blinding reviewers and asking them to sign their reports: a randomised controlled trial. *JAMA* 1998;**280**:237–40.

9 Van Royen S, Godlee F, Evans S, Smith R, Black N. Effect of blinding and unmasking on the quality of peer review: a randomised controlled trial. *JAMA* 1998;**280**:234–7.

10 Godlee F. Making reviewers visible. Openness, accountability, and credit. *JAMA* 2002;**287**:2762–5.

11 Smith R. Opening up *BMJ* peer review. *BMJ* 1999;**318**:4–5.

12 Callaham ML, Knopp RK, Gallagher EJ. Effect of written feedback by editors on quality of reviews. *JAMA* 2002;**287**:2781–3.

13 Schroter S, Black N, Evans S, Smith R, Carpenter J, Godlee F. Effects of training on the quality of peer review: a randomised controlled trial. *BMJ* 2004;**328**:673–5.

14 Schroter S, Groves T. BMJ training for peer reviewers. *BMJ* 2004;**328**:658.

15 Black N, van Rooyen S, Godlee F, Smith R, Evans S. What makes a good reviewer and a good review in a general medical journal. *JAMA* 1998;**280**:231–3.

16 Weber EJ, Katz PP, Waeckerle JF, Callaham MI. Author perception of peer review. *JAMA* 2002;**287**:2790–3.

17 Smith R. Misconduct in research: editors respond. *BMJ* 1997;**315**:201–2.

Chapter 15 **What a publisher does**

Alex Williamson

Congratulations! Your paper has been accepted for publication.

At this point, the author may have his or her first contact with the publisher. This should be a rewarding and pleasant experience, but many authors have only a vague notion of what a publisher actually does.

Authors write and the publishers provide the means for those authors to reach their audiences – traditionally via a print medium. Now we also have the means to reach a potentially much larger and more international audience via the Internet – on average the online audience is at least three times larger than the print circulation. The services that a journal publishing house offers fall into a number of broad categories: editorial, production, sales and marketing, subscription fulfilment, distribution, and finance. An author will have no direct contact with some of the latter categories, but they nevertheless are essential to the business. Each category is dependent on the others, and all work closely together.

Editorial

Typically three main functions exist within the editorial department – managing, commissioning, and copy editing. In many cases the publisher also takes responsibility for managing the administration of the manuscript submission and peer review process. In other cases the learned society or the editors themselves take on this task.

Managing and commissioning editors

Managing and commissioning editors (also called publishing managers, acquisitions editors, or sponsoring editors) are the publishers' representatives to journal editors, learned societies, and authors. The main function of a managing editor is the care of the existing list of journals. This consists of financial management, liaison with the learned society (if one is involved), overseeing the duties of the copy editor, editorial assistants, both online and print production, advertisement sales, marketing, subscription fulfilment and distribution, and – last but by no means least – liaison with and support of the journal editors. These editors are a rare breed of dedicated professionals who are often full time clinicians, academics, or both. For modest or no reward, they devote many hours to editorial work and need strong support from the publisher.

Managing editors will also receive new journal proposals, seek specialist opinion via both questionnaires and personal contacts, analyse and research the market, cost the proposal, and, finally, present it to their management. The rejection rate for new journal proposals is very high indeed – roughly speaking, only one in 10 proposals will be successful. A new journal launch requires a large investment from the publisher, so a decision to launch is never taken lightly.

The managing editor will meet the editor regularly, offer advice on publishing practice, and help to train support staff for the editorial office. In recent times, the managing editor has had to learn a new skill: they need to be up to date with Internet developments.

More than 90% of scientific, technical, and medical journals now have an online presence as well as a print version. Most journals' online versions have now evolved into very sophisticated sites, with html and pdf full text, search engines, substantial back archives, subject collections, data supplements, blogs and pod casts, videos, email alerts, rapid responses, 'online firsts', hyperlinks to other useful sites, RSS feeds and much, much more. The managing editor should be able to recommend new functionalities, suggest the uploading of additional data to enhance the site, and make it a much more useful and comprehensive resource than the print version. An increasing number of journals now regard the online as the definitive version and the print product merely a subset of what is available online.

The whole peer review process has also undergone significant change in recent times. The Internet has revolutionised the peer review process, and the signs are that it is speeding it up too. Most journals have migrated to a web-based manuscript submission and peer review system. This means that the journal is 'open for business' 24h a day, 7 days a week, and it is accessible from anywhere in the world that has Internet access. It is now almost irrelevant as to where the editorial office is situated. Indeed, there are journals where the editor is in one country, the editorial assistant in another and the publisher's office in a third. Despite this revolution, the editorial assistant is still a key player. He or she ensures that manuscripts are kept moving through the system, assists authors who have uploading problems, chases recalcitrant authors and reviewers (and editors), acts as editorial secretary and gives general administrative support to the editorial team. Usually these assistants are recruited, funded and trained by the publisher and are full-time employees but may be freelances working from home. The whole process has been streamlined and is more cost effective and efficient but inevitably some sacrifices have been made. There are some editors, reviewers, and authors who criticise the impersonality of these web-based systems – no more wonderfully crafted personal rejection letters signed with the editor's quill pen! It is also true that a reviewer receiving an impersonal email soliciting a review is more inclined to press 'no' than they were when a large courier delivered package thumped onto their desk with a personal letter from the editor politely asking for an opinion. These systems also seem to have increased the number of submissions to journals and have certainly broken down the barriers that used to exist for some overseas authors whose postal services left much to be desired.

Once a manuscript is accepted for publication, the editor or editorial assistant will send it as an electronic file to the publisher, where it will receive the attention of the copy editor.

Copy editors

Copy editors (also called technical editors, subeditors, or production editors) provide the main link between an author and the publisher. The copy editor will prepare the accepted manuscript for publication in print and on the web. Most copy editing is now done on screen using the author's own word processed file. These author files are now often passed through some editing software that will clean up the file and apply styles prior to the copy editor starting work. Copy editors have learned new skills and, in many cases, will be adding tagging and codes to the word processed author file so that the page make up programme can operate seamlessly and take in the artwork, figures, and tables, which will also have been generated electronically. The copy editor will also scrutinise the tables and illustrations.

Copy editors adapt the manuscript to the 'house style' of the journal and ensure that the author has complied with the journal's instructions. They are concerned with details of style and ensure that spelling, grammar, punctuation, capitalisation, and mathematical conventions follow approved practice. They also look for accuracy and consistency. They pick up loose ends, discrepancies, omissions, and contradictions. Substantive queries may be referred back to the author and editor at this stage. More often, the problems identified are minor and will appear as queries to the author on the proof. Copy editors will suggest relettering and redrawing of illustrations where necessary and will size them and place them appropriately in the text. Their edited files will then be translated automatically into the appropriate format for the print and electronic versions of the journal.

Copy editors liaise with the supplier and ensure that proofs are distributed quickly to authors and editors. They will read the proofs and collate any corrections received from authors and editors. Only in exceptional circumstances are authors allowed to make major changes to their papers at this stage, and the copy editor will refer substantive author corrections for the editor's approval.

Copy editors work to tight schedules and often need to remind authors to return proofs promptly. Again, technology is helping to speed up the process. Many publishers require their suppliers to provide proofs in a pdf format, so that they can be emailed to authors as an attachment.

In collaboration with the editor and the advertisement department, copy editors make up the contents of each issue and pass final proofs for press. At this stage, the publishing process passes to the production department.

In many publishing houses, copy editors are often freelances working from home or the service may be out sourced overseas. In these cases, after editing, the journal make up and further liaison with the editor is provided by the publishers' in house production editors.

Again, the Internet has speeded up the publication process. Many journals now offer an 'online first' service. On acceptance either a pdf of the final accepted but unedited manuscript is put online immediately or it is put online after the copy editing process. When the print issue is published the final formatted and edited version overlays the earlier version that was posted. This means that a paper can be published and indexed by PubMed within a day or two of acceptance whereas the print version may not appear for another 3–6 months, or longer. Authors, of course, love this! One molecular biology title boasts of a decision within 24 h and posting online the same day if the paper is accepted without further revision.

Copyright

Either at acceptance of the manuscript for publication or at the proof stage, the author may be required to assign copyright to the journal. Publishers are much better able to defend copyright than individual authors and will act on their behalf. However, practices are changing. Now, many journals simply require that authors grant them an exclusive licence to publish their article in print and on the web. Authors retain copyright and are able to use their own material freely elsewhere. Many authors are now requested or mandated by their research funders to deposit the accepted manuscript or final published version in a subject-based repository such as PubMedCentral or their own institutional repository. Many publishers will allow this but may require an embargo period of anything from 6 to 24 months to safeguard the journal's subscription business model.

Offprints

Offprints are extra copies of the articles that are printed at the same time as the journal issue. Some publishers offer a quantity of these gratis to the author. This used to be a very popular service for authors, but the ease of photocopying has almost eliminated the need. Many publishers have now substituted provision of a free copy of the relevant journal issue to the corresponding author instead of providing free offprints. Other publishers will offer the author the opportunity to purchase a quantity of reprints at cost. In addition, some journals provide a pdf of the article to the author or free access to that article on the journal's website.

Production

Very few journals now use conventional typesetters, instead, edited electronic files are sent to an originating house (sometimes this may be a part of a major printing house). Here the edited text files are married with the tables, figures, and illustrations, and the article is proofed. After final approval for publication and the journal issue has been made up, the online and print versions take different routes.

The print production staff will choose appropriate printers for the journal, bearing in mind the budget, print run, schedule, and use of colour illustrations and advertisements. They choose and purchase text paper and cover boards. The production department is responsible for schedules, obtains estimates, and controls costs. It keeps abreast of the latest advances in print and bind technology, and it will advise editorial colleagues on appropriate new means of production that will benefit the journal in terms of schedule, cost, and appearance. Overall, the production team is responsible for the look of the journal, its cost effective production on schedule, and its delivery for onward distribution to subscribers.

Most publishers have chosen a third party for hosting and maintaining their journal websites. On completion of an issue, the electronic files are sent to the hosting service for the addition of further programming before uploading. Many journal websites also have sections that are under the control of the editor and publisher to facilitate the addition of extra material and hyperlinks on a daily basis.

Fulfilment and distribution

The average peer reviewed journal's circulation is subscription based, usually on an annual basis. Again, the availability of online versions of most journals has given more options but undoubtedly has made the entire process more complex. Some publishers 'bundle' their subscriptions so customers pay a single price and receive both a print version and access to the online version. Others have 'unbundled' and offer a choice between print or online versions. All manner of pricing models exist based on simultaneous users, tiers depending on institutional size, print deeply discounted if online is taken and so on. Increasingly too, publishers will offer online site licences for all their titles to libraries or consortias of libraries, often at deep discounts – the so-called 'Big Deal'. This has had quite a bad press and most publishers will allow their customers to 'pick and mix'. Librarians now have good usage statistics for their holdings and journals that aren't used get cancelled.

By and large, subscribers fall into four main categories:

1 Institutional or library subscriptions at the full price subscription rate. Most of these sales are handled via subscription agents, who make the librarians' jobs much simpler. Librarians will probably deal with only one agent for the thousands of subscriptions they purchase. The agent will consolidate these orders and deal with the individual publishers, quite often using computers to facilitate the transfer of orders. For this service, most publishers give agents a discount.

2 Personal subscriptions at a discounted subscription rate.

3 Member subscriptions. Often a journal will be owned by or published in association with a learned society. The annual membership subscription may include an automatic subscription to the society's journal.

4 Free and exchange subscriptions. The editor and editorial board will normally receive free copies. Copyright legislation decrees that journal issues must be deposited in the British Library and several other major libraries. Subscriptions are given to the large abstracting and indexing services such as *Index Medicus* also known as *PubMed*, *Current Contents*, and *Scopus*.

All of these groups expect to receive the journal regularly and on time, and subscribers need to be reminded each year to renew their subscriptions. Most subscription fulfilment systems are computer based and will generate mailing labels sorted into postal categories to a defined schedule. In many cases, these mailing labels will be despatched directly to the printer, who will arrange onward posting to subscribers. In other cases, publishers will handle all distribution from their own warehouses. Overseas consignments are often sent in bulk by air to a mailing house, which then organises onward distribution by that country's mail service. The warehouse will store additional copies of the journal to fulfil claims for missing issues, back orders, and single copy sales.

Sales and marketing

The main source of revenue for the majority of journals comes from the sale of paid subscriptions. There are other sources, however, and I will deal with these before returning to the subscription area.

Advertising sales

The higher circulation general and specialist clinical journals enjoy substantial revenues from the sale of display and classified advertising space in each issue. The major space buyers are the pharmaceutical companies, but equipment manufacturers, conference and event organisers and publishers also use journals to advertise their products.

The advertisement sales team not only maintains close links with agencies and companies, but it also liaises with the editorial team. A strong editorial policy on the percentage of advertisement versus editorial pages is needed, together with a strict code on the permitted content of advertisements and their location in comparison with editorial pages. Many journals operate a strict policy of not allowing advertisement sales in relation to editorial copy, and often editors will be allowed the right of veto. Despite these safeguards, editors, and publishers are often criticised about the content and placement of advertisements. Nevertheless, advertisements can provide a useful service to the reader and certainly support the journal financially. The sale of advertising space to online versions is still in its infancy, and whilst it has become very successful in other areas, it is fair to say that at least outside the United States, it has not delivered substantial revenue streams to European publishers yet.

Reprint sales

Reprint sales can be a considerable source of revenue, particularly where papers are reporting the results of clinical trials or new indications for an existing drug. They are usually in bulk, are of necessity more expensive than offprints, and appeal to the commercial sector, particularly the pharmaceutical industry who rely on giving them to potential prescribers as a key part of their marketing campaigns. Some journals claim higher revenues from reprint sales than from the sale of print subscriptions and online site licenses.

Rights

The marketing of a journal involves not only the sale of subscriptions but also the sale of subsidiary rights. These may take the form of translation rights, rights to produce an English language edition in a slightly modified form for a foreign market, or rights to produce cheap reprints in countries where purchasing power is low. Additionally, journals will sell the rights to host their content or header information to third-party aggregators such as Ovid or Ingenta. Digital rights management has become the vogue and many journal websites now incorporate software that enables the user to seek permission to reuse the content and pay online.

Bulk and single copy sales and online sales

Occasionally, a journal will publish a special issue or supplement on a particular 'hot' topic, and this may attract bulk sales from a commercial organisation or single copy sales to individuals. Many journal websites also carry 'pay per view' or 'pay for access'. This functionality facilitated by e-commerce packages allows non-subscribers to access particular articles or to have access to the whole site for a period for payment of a modest sum.

Subscription sales and marketing

When a new journal is launched, the circulation climbs steadily and then plateaus as the journal becomes established in its specialty. Some people are of the opinion that once a journal has reached its plateau, it is no longer necessary to continue active promotion. Not so! Every year, an established journal will lose some 10% of its circulation because of consolidation of library collections, budgetary restrictions, or simply a change in the direction of research in the institution.

To maintain its circulation, a journal needs to be promoted to pick up new subscribers to replace those that have been lost. In collaboration with the subscription and fulfilment department, the lapsed subscribers will be encouraged actively to renew their subscriptions, and ultimately they will receive a questionnaire that can provide valuable information to editorial colleagues.

The marketing department is concerned with promotion material, publicity, and advertising. It devises campaigns to promote each journal, and it designs, writes, and produces leaflets and catalogues that are sent by direct mail to specialists and librarians worldwide. Apart from direct mail, journals are promoted via advertisements in other relevant high-circulation journals and displays at appropriate specialty meetings and symposia.

As in every other facet of publishing, the Internet also has changed the role of the marketing executive. Although most of the activities outlined above continue, often in a lesser form, the marketeers' role has changed to promoting usage of the website and attracting new authors and readers. All but the very small publishers now have an international sales force that has face-to-face contacts with their customers – usually institutional librarians or representatives of the major consortia (groups of libraries that come together to increase their buying power). Some publishers now host library advisory groups where publisher and librarian can exchange views and take heed of each others' needs.

The Internet is now used as a very effective marketing tool that can reach a large target audience very cheaply, and, if managed well, it can provide useful details of the customers who visit the site. Most of the major publishers have websites that act as a showcase for their publications. Many of these sites will also enable e-commerce so that orders can be placed and paid for directly. Targeted email campaigns seem more effective than relying on the old stalwart of direct mail shots.

Finance

The members of staff of the finance department have a number of roles – all of them concerned with money! They raise invoices, control cash flow, maintain records, and pay suppliers. The management accountant will provide monthly accounts to the senior management and will play an integral part in the construction of annual budgets and ensuring they are met, and longer-term strategic planning.

Conclusion

The role of the publisher has been compared with a variety of functions, few of them favourable. We have been told we are parasites or denigrated as middlemen who come between the author and the reader. Perhaps we are best regarded as catalysts. We facilitate the communication between the authors and their readers. Even with the arrival of the Internet, we are still needed to provide an efficient means to sift through, sort, and disseminate the fruits of your labours. Of late, publishers have enjoyed a bad press with the continued rise of the 'Open Access' movement. It is true that the movement has had a particularly effective PR machine and publishers have not responded as well as they might. However, many journals now offer open access choices for authors and some titles have gone over completely to open access. Many journals, particularly society-owned titles make all their content freely accessible online after 6, 12, or 24 months.

Nevertheless, the fact remains that as long as the peer reviewed journal continues to be the *lingua franca* of academic achievement and the means of dissemination of scientific and clinical research, journals and their publishers will continue to exist as the owners, investors, and guardians of the scientific record.

Chapter 16 **Who should be an author?**

Richard Horton

Regrettably this question is impossible to answer. Ten years ago, I could have confidently referred you to the standard definition provided by the International Committee of Medical Journal Editors (otherwise known as the Vancouver Group) (Box 16.1) [1]. All was clear back then. The criteria that had to be satisfied for you to qualify as an author (to be, shall we say, Vancouver Group positive) were unambiguous.

And they needed to be. Authorship is the currency of academic life. Citation provides the intellectual credit that fuels promotion and career success; it gives an independent estimate of a researcher's contribution to science. Authorship is the foundation of our system for judging academic value and assigning reward.

Before I ruin this picture of serene harmony, I should point out that most biomedical journals adhere to the Vancouver Group definition [2]. Their editors will require you to be Vancouver Group positive. In other words, to confirm in either a covering letter or a separate signed statement that you fulfil the Vancouver definition. You are likely to say you do even if you know that you or a co-author does not. To provide your signature confirming that you qualify as an author is something you do automatically, perhaps without even thinking very much about the implications of what you are doing.

Nowadays, though, the certainty that editors of leading medical journals once possessed lies in shreds. Our happy consensus has been destroyed. Following a conference on authorship in biomedical science, held in Nottingham, UK, in 1996 [3], first the *Lancet* [4] and then the *BMJ* [5] abandoned the Vancouver Group definition (although their editors are part of the Group). In its place we put the concept of contributorship, an idea first described by Fotion and Conrad [6] but developed more fully by Drummond Rennie and colleagues [7,8]. This shift away from traditional notions of authorship is the most important recent crack to appear in the architecture of academia. It has the potential to threaten the entire structure of modern science. Why? And where does that leave you, someone who simply wants to get your work published?

Box 16.1 How to be a Vancouver Group positive author

All persons designated as authors should qualify for authorship. Each author should have participated sufficiently in the work to take public responsibility for the content.

Authorship credit should be based only on substantial contributions to: (1) conception and design or analysis and interpretation of data; (2) drafting the article or revising it critically for important intellectual content; and (3) final approval of the version to be published. Conditions 1–3 must all be met. Participation solely in the acquisition of funding or the collection of data does not justify authorship. General supervision of the research group is not sufficient for authorship. Any part of an article critical to its main conclusions must be the responsibility of at least one author.

Editors may ask authors to describe what each contributed; this information may be published.

Increasingly, multicentre trials are attributed to a corporate author. All members of the group who are named as authors, either in the authorship position below the title or in a footnote, should fully meet the above criteria for authorship. Group members who do not meet: these criteria should be listed, with their permission, in the acknowledgements or in an appendix.

The order of authorship should be a joint decision of the co-authors. Because the order is assigned in different ways, its meaning cannot be inferred accurately unless it is stated by the authors. Authors may wish to explain the order of authorship in a footnote. In deciding on the order, authors should be aware that many journals limit the number of authors listed in the table of contents and that the US National Library of Medicine (NLM) lists in Medline only the first 24 plus the last author when there are more than 25 authors.

First, most scientists ignore editors and most so-called authors are likely to test Vancouver Group negative. For example, Shapiro *et al.* [9] found that a quarter of the 'authors' they surveyed contributed nothing or to only one aspect of the published work.

Eastwood *et al.* [10] discovered that a third of the US postdoctoral fellows they questioned were happy to list someone as an author even if he or she did not deserve it, provided that the inclusion of their name would make publication more likely. Given this widespread cynicism about the meaning of authorship, to cling to a definition that no one uses seems crazy.

There is a second, more sensitive reason for questioning our existing beliefs about authorship. Several recent instances of scientific fraud [11,12] have revealed that the flipside of authorship *credit* – namely, authorship *responsibility* – is often overlooked. When individual researchers have their names listed on the byline of a paper, it can be difficult to dissect out who did what if an aspect of the work is questioned. Instances of fabrication or falsification of data have revealed the importance of assigning the precise and explicit parts played by individual investigators in a research project.

These two forces make it hard to resist two ensuing interpretations. First, researchers should be allowed to list whoever they wish on the byline of a paper, Vancouver Group positive or negative. And second, editors should ask for and publish a clear description of the contributions made by the authors. Rigid, unenforceable, and widely ignored definitions should be abandoned. This is the new policy of the *BMJ* [5] and the *Lancet* [4]. The *BMJ* has gone further than the *Lancet* and asks each group of contributors to select one or more guarantors who will take overall responsibility for the integrity of the entire work.

The reaction to contributorship has been mixed. At the *Lancet*, we have found that most authors readily accept the idea that contributors should be cited at the end of each paper (Box 16.2). But some have voiced concerns that unethical authorship practices – inappropriate credit in the form of guest authors or the unacknowledged contributions of ghost authors – are likely to continue [13].

Box 16.2 An example of contributorship

Byline: A, B, C, D, E, F, G, H
Contributors: A carried out the trial, helped in data analysis, and wrote the paper. B was involved in design, implementation, and data analysis, and contributed to the writing of the paper. C was involved in execution of the trial, data management and analysis, and quality assurance of the turnip assay. D was involved in trial execution and data entry, management analysis, and quality assurance. E was involved in trial execution and data management with emphasis on analysis. F and G were involved in the design and contributed to the writing of the paper. H was involved in the design, implementation, analysis, and biochemical interpretation, and contributed to the writing of the paper.
Guarantors: A and H

Still, other journals are likely to follow the move to contributorship. Even if contributor lists are not always embraced, the principle of complete disclosure and personal responsibility is accepted [14]. You need to be aware which journals prefer traditional Vancouver Group positive authors and which prefer contributors. For all practical purposes, you can freely ignore the rules set by the former group. Everybody else does.

An additional issue that also defies easy rules is the acknowledgement section of your paper. Whom you choose to thank can be impossible to separate from whom you choose to cite as an author on the byline. Not surprisingly, the Vancouver Group has something to say about acknowledgements (Box 16.3). The likelihood is that contributor lists and acknowledgements will eventually fuse and the whole subject of academic reward based on research contributions will be overhauled [15].

Box 16.3 Acknowledgements according to Vancouver

At an appropriate place in the article (the title page footnote or an appendix to the text; see the journal's requirements), one or more statements should specify: (1) contributions that need acknowledging but do not justify authorship, such as general support by a departmental chair; (2) acknowledgements of technical help; (3) acknowledgements of financial and material support, which should specify the nature of the support; and (4) relationships that may pose a conflict of interest.

Persons who have contributed intellectually to the paper but whose contributions do not justify authorship may be named and their function or contribution described – for example, 'scientific adviser', 'critical review of study proposal', 'data collection', or 'participation in clinical trial'. Such persons must have given their permission to be named. Authors are responsible for obtaining written permission from persons acknowledged by name, because readers may infer their endorsement of the data and conclusions.

Technical help should be acknowledged in a paragraph separate from that acknowledging other contributions.

Given this confusing state, there is only one rule to bear in mind when deciding who is an author, a contributor, a guarantor, or an acknowledgee. Decide who is to be what before you start your study. Most authorship disputes arise when the work is completed and a paper has to be written. Then comes the jostling for a place (and position) on the byline. Primary prevention is always better in the end.

References

1 International Committee of Medical Journal Editors. Uniform requirements for manuscripts submitted to biomedical journals. *Ann Intern Med* 1997;**126**:36–47.
2 Parmley WW. Authorship: taking the high road. *J Am Coll Cardiol* 1997;**29**:702.
3 Horton R, Smith R. Signing up for authorship. *Lancet* 1996;**347**:780.
4 Horton R. The signature of responsibility. *Lancet* 1997;**350**:5–6.
5 Smith R. Authorship is dying: long live contributorship. *BMJ* 1997; **315**:686.

6 Fotion N, Conrad CC. Authorship and other credits. *Ann Intern Med* 1984; **100**: 592–4.

7 Rennie D, Flanagin A. Authorship! Authorship! Guests, ghosts, grafters, and the two-sided coin. *JAMA* 1994; **278**: 469–71.

8 Rennie D, Yank V, Emanuel L. When authorship fails: a proposal to make contributors accountable. *JAMA* 1997; **278**: 579–85.

9 Shapiro SW, Wenger NS, Shapiro ME. The contributions of authors to multiauthored biomedical research papers. *JAMA* 1994; **271**: 438–42.

10 Eastwood S, Derish P, Leash E, Ordway S. Ethical issues in biomedical research: perceptions and practices of postdoctoral research fellows responding to a survey. *Sci Eng Ethics* 1996; **2**: 89–114.

11 Lock S. Lessons from the Pearce affair: handling scientific fraud. *BMJ* 1995; **310**: 1547–8.

12 Marshall E. Fraud strikes top genome lab. *Science* 1996; **274**: 908–10.

13 Greenfield B, Kaufman JL, Hueston WJ, Mainous AG, De Bakey L, DeBakey S. Authors vs contributors: accuracy, accountability, and responsibility. *JAMA* 1998; **279**: 356–7.

14 Editorial. Games people play with authors' names. *Nature* 1997; **387**: 831.

15 Horton R. The unmasked carnival of science. *Lancet* 1998; **351**: 688–9.

Chapter 17 **Style: what it is and why it matters**

Margaret Cooter

The first step towards producing a 'stylish' paper is good organisation of the contents, and the preceding chapters have dealt with gathering the information you need and structuring your article. The next step is good writing – good scientific style. A further step, house style, will be added by the journal's editorial staff.

A scientific article needs to be fit for its purpose, which is the communication of information. When drafting or revising your paper, you need to keep three main things in mind:

- be clear,
- be accurate,
- be concise.

Clarity

Authors of scientific papers are so familiar with their subject that they risk being unclear to their readers. Each specialty has its buzzwords and jargon – but the language of medical conversation often isn't appropriate for clear communication with readers from outside the specialty or for readers whose first language isn't English.

By paying attention to grammar and punctuation, and by choosing words carefully, you will communicate more clearly.

- Give readers the information they need in a convenient order and in manageable chunks.
- Define terms, such as abbreviations and jargon, that may be unfamiliar to readers.
- Use the right word – if you doubt it for an instant, check the word's meaning in a dictionary. Beware of easily confused words, like mitigate and militate.
- Use sentences with simple clear structures. These are likely to be short sentences.

- Jargon should be reserved for specialist contexts. In general writing, avoiding jargon will help you express ideas simply and directly.
- Noun clusters can be confusing – 'spell them out' by adding appropriate prepositions: child abuse allegations = allegations of child abuse; speed reduction measures = measures to reduce speed; obstetric complication frequency = frequency of obstetric complications.
- Use the active rather than the passive voice. Say who did what: we compared the treatment group with the control group (*Note*: The treatment and control groups were compared). Although traditional teaching is to use the passive voice in scientific articles, readers prefer active sentences, and so do many journals.
- Try not to start sentences with 'there is' or 'there are' – this is a deadening phrase. Usually, changing the verb will let you get rid of 'there is' – and make the sentence active.

   'There is a report on the two programmes' is less dull when changed to 'A report on the two programmes is available'.
- Make sure the verbs are in the right tense and agree with the noun they refer to:

   Strengthening the capacities to deal with these problems in developing countries is important (is, not are: the verb refers to 'strengthening', not 'capacities' or 'countries').
- When you use the word this, these, they, he, she, or it, be sure that exactly what, or who, the word refers to is clear. This sentence needs changing:

   If the baby does not thrive on raw milk, boil it.
- Make comparisons clear – don't assume that readers will know which two (or more) things are being compared. This is important when there are several possibilities – for example, is the comparison with another subgroup or is it with the whole population? In some cases, the comparison is dichotomous, and the comparator need not be stated:

   More women [than men] were alive five years after diagnosis.
- Careful punctuation avoids ambiguity. Know the difference between defining clauses (no comma) and commenting clauses (commas needed):

   Medical staff who often work overtime are likely to suffer from stress.
   Medical staff, who often work overtime, are likely to suffer from stress.

Accuracy

When you are adding to the body of knowledge, you don't want mistakes in your paper, or to give scope for misunderstandings.
- Use scientific conventions (SI units, symbols, Greek letters) correctly.
- Give numbers as well as percentages in results – and check your arithmetic.

- Use, but don't rely on, a spell checker – it won't tell you that a 'not' is missing from your sentence.
- Check that names are spelt correctly.
- Check that reference numbers (if you are using the Vancouver system) refer to the correct reference in the reference list, and that they are in sequence in the text.
- Check that all tables and figures are referred to in the text, and that the same terms are used within the figure as are used in the figure legend.

Conciseness

Simply by being clear and accurate, you are well on the way to saying what you have to say in the briefest way possible.

- Good structure and organisation will keep the paper 'tight'.
- Use the simple word rather than the irritating pomposity: before (not 'prior to'); more than (not 'in excess of'); depends on (not 'is dependent upon'); also (not 'additionally'); too (not 'overly'); indicates (not 'is indicative of').
- Avoid phrases like 'it is well known that'.
- Avoid clichés – are they actually saying anything important?
- Keep an eye out for tautology – for example, 'a prior history'.

Critical review

When you have written and rewritten, stand back from your manuscript – put it away for a few days and then re-read it critically. Better yet, ask a trusted colleague to review it and point out anything that is ambiguous or unclear.

House style

The journal to which you submit your manuscript may supply, or have available on its website, a style sheet that sets out some basic decisions the editors have made to get consistency in layout, punctuation, capitalisation, terminology, and so on throughout the journal. For example, guidance in the *BMJ's* 'Essentials of style' (http://bmj.com/advice/stylebook/basics.shtml) includes:

- *Minimal hyphenation*: Use hyphens only for words with non-, -like, -type, and for adjectival phrases that include a preposition (one-off event, run-in trial). Not using hyphens will help you to avoid noun clusters.
- *Minimal capitalisation*: Use capitals only for names and proper nouns. Don't capitalise names of studies.
- *Quotation marks*: Use double, not single, inverted commas for reported speech. Full stops and commas go inside quotation marks.

- *Sex*: Avoid 'he' as a general pronoun. Make the nouns (and pronouns) plural, then use 'they'; if that's not possible, use 'he or she'.
- *Use English, not American spelling*: Aetiology, oestradiol, anaemia, haemorrhage, practice (noun), practise (verb). Foetus and fetus are both acceptable in English: the *BMJ* uses fetus.
- Drugs should be referred to by their approved non-proprietary names, and the source of any new or experimental preparations should be given.

The style book used by the *BMJ's* technical editors elaborates on these, and similar, points. It also contains a plethora of specific decisions that have had to be made – and revised – over many decades: Antimalaria drugs or antimalarial drugs? Capitalise job titles, or not – the Director General or the director general? When are abbreviations allowed? Beta-carotene or β carotene? Moslem or Muslim; Myanmar or Burma?

Some of the principles of house style are standards of good writing; others are admittedly arbitrary, but these provide consistency throughout the publication and help to give a journal its identity (Box 17.1).

Box 17.1 Style makes a difference

- Good style assists effective communication
- Style should aid, not hinder, comprehension
- Clear writing helps articles be accepted for publication
- Well-presented papers make editors' jobs easier
- House style gives publications consistency and identity

Your proofs

Even the best writers will find changes on their proofs. This is because the journal's editorial staff will have gone through the paper to deal with possible ambiguity and to implement house style.

Technical editors (also known as copy editors or subeditors) serve as the reader's advocate, focusing on areas that a reader would find unclear or redundant. Through their exacting scrutiny of papers before publication, technical editors aim to remove the obstacles that would hinder a reader's easy grasp of the message and details of the paper, while not distorting what the author has to say.

Towards this goal technical editors ensure that:

- the paper is free of errors of spelling and grammar (unclear antecedents, misplaced modifiers, and subject–verb agreement problems account for 80% or more of these);
- the paper's structure is clear – this may require rewording, reorganisation, adding headings, or writing transitions;

- sentences that are unclear, and unsupported conclusions or gaps in logic, are pointed out to the author on the proof or discussed before proof stage;
- jargon is eliminated or explained, so that readers unfamiliar with the speciality will grasp the meaning;
- verbosity is eliminated;
- names are spelt consistently (and correctly);
- acronyms and abbreviations are defined or spelt out on first use and used in accordance with house style throughout the paper;
- arithmetic (totals in columns of tables; numbers and percentages) is correct.

Technical editors will also 'tag' the paper for electronic production, and your proof may look different from the final, published format because of this.

Smooth your paper's path to publication

Make the editor's job easier – and speed your paper on its way to publication – by learning what you can about the journal's style requirements. Be sure to look at the journal's guidelines for authors or its advice to contributors, and include all the elements that are specified in the guidelines.

- Check the journal's style sheet, if there is one – it may be sent to you when your paper is accepted subject to revision, it may be published in the journal at intervals, or detailed guidance may be available on the journal's website.
- Make sure your 'title page' contains all the elements published in the journal – addresses, affiliations, job titles, corresponding author, and keywords.
- Return all the necessary forms with your revised article (e.g. copyright assignment, competing interests, and permissions); the editor will need to have these so that, in the interests of transparency, statements of funding or competing interests can be added to the article.
- Respond fully to the editor's queries on the proof. Changes have been made because something was unclear, so don't just reinstate your original wording.
- Editors are only human and do make mistakes – if the editor's changes distort your meaning, do point this out.

Further reading

Guides to writing

Albert T, ed. *The A–Z of medical writing*. London: BMJ Books, 2000.

Carey JV. *Mind the stop: a brief guide to punctuation*. London: Penguin, 1976.

Fowler H, Winchester S. *Fowler's modern English usage*. Oxford: Oxford University Press, 2002.

Goodman NW, Edwards ME. *Medical writing: a prescription for clarity*, 2nd edn. Cambridge: Cambridge University Press, 1997.

Greenbaum S, Whitcut J. *Longman guide to English usage*. London: Penguin, 1996.

Kirkman J. *Good style: writing for science and technology*. London: E&FN Spon, 1992.

O'Connor M. *Writing successfully in science*. London: Chapman & Hall, 1999.

Strunk Jr W, White EB. *The elements of style*. Boston: Allyn & Bacon, 1999.

Style manuals

American Medical Association. *Manual of style: a guide for authors and editors*, 9th edn. Philadelphia: Lippincott Williams & Wilkins, 1998.

BMJ house style. http://bmj.com/advice/stylebook/start.shtml

Council of Biology Editors. *Scientific style and format*, 6th edn. New York: Cambridge University Press, 1994.

Chapter 18 **Ethics of publication**

Michael J.G. Farthing

Introduction

The world of science is totally dependent on the integrity of those involved in all aspects of the research and publishing process. Investigators and research students, authors, peer reviewers, and journal editors must operate within an ethical framework, which is totally transparent and has principles that are understood and accepted by all players in the biomedical research community. Ethical considerations have taken centre stage in the protection of the rights of patients and healthy volunteers in clinical research and in considering the welfare of animals used in biomedical research.

There is a growing concern that research misconduct has become more frequent during the past two decades. It is difficult to be certain whether this perceived increase is a true increase in the number of misdemeanours committed, but there is no doubt that the number of serious cases of research misconduct that have been detected has increased during this period. As editor of a specialist journal, I saw many examples of research and publication misconduct [1,2]. Stephen Lock, a past editor of the *BMJ*, has documented known or suspected cases of research misconduct in the United Kingdom, the United States, Australia, Canada, and other countries [3].

Research misconduct in biomedicine has been brought sharply into focus because of the recent high-profile cases reported from North America, Southeast Asia, and Europe during the last 2 or 3 years. Dr Eric Poehlman for example, who was a senior researcher into the menopause, ageing, and metabolism at the University of Vermont, was forced to retract 10 major publications in high impact factor journals and was also found to have fabricated data in many grant applications. He lost his job, was fined $250,000 and faces a law suit [4]. Luk van Parijs working on RNA silencing at MIT was also subject to allegations of serious research misconduct, which eventually resulted in the loss of his job in 2005 [5]. Perhaps the most recent high-profile case is that of Professor Hwang in South Korea which resulted in the retraction of several papers from major scientific journals, loss of his job, and termination of a relationship with Korean Airlines which gave him and his family free first class flights around the world. He may also face a court case for research fraud [6,7]. Research misconduct is not limited to medicine and biomedical science; there have been investigations of misconduct in physics, ecology, and nano-electronics in recent years [8–10].

What is publication ethics?

It is vital that scientists engaged in biomedical research should be fully informed of the ethical framework in which they should be operating. The Committee on Publication Ethics (COPE) published guidelines on Good Publication Practice in 1999 [11] and continues to update these on a regular basis (http://www.publicationethics.org.uk). These guidelines cover a range of issues including study design and ethical approval, data analysis and presentation, authorship, conflicts of interest, peer review, redundant publication, duties of editors, media relations, advertising and research misconduct.

Study design
A poorly designed study unable to answer the research question posed should be regarded as unethical. The design of the study – including patient numbers, controls, experimental methods, and data analysis, etc. – should all be clearly articulated in a written protocol. In clinical studies, power calculations should be performed to ensure that the number of subjects to be included in the study will be large enough to give a definitive result. Failure to do this can be regarded as unethical. If doubt exists about the power of a study, take specialised advice; it is usually too late to do this as part of a rescue procedure at the end of the study. Local research ethics committees may withhold ethical approval until shortcomings in study design have been rectified. The final protocol should be agreed by all investigators and their contributions clearly defined [12]. It is much safer to agree the authorship of any papers that might emerge from the study at this early stage to avoid later disputes.

Ethical approval
Approval from an appropriately constituted research ethics committee is mandatory for all studies involving people, medical records, and anonymised human tissues. When study participants are unable to give fully informed consent, the research protocol should adhere closely to international guidelines, such as those of the Council for International Organisations of Medical Sciences (CIOMS). In recent years, the ethical standards for the use of human

tissues in biomedical research have increased. If human tissues or body fluids have been collected for one project for which ethical approval and consent was obtained, it cannot be assumed that these archived samples can be used again without further consent. Many countries now attempt to minimise the number of animals used in biomedical research. It should be assumed that no journal will publish human or animal studies that do not conform to the ethical standards of the country in which the journal is published.

Regular reviews of research findings should be made, including examination of the original research records. Any protocol changes during the course of the study should be agreed by all investigators. Original research records should be retained for 15 years by the institution in which the work was carried out.

Data analysis

The approach to data analysis should be clearly stated in the protocol; deviations such as *post hoc* analyses and/or data exclusion should be agreed by all investigators and disclosed in the paper. The potential now to electronically manipulate data – particularly images such as immunoblots, gels, audioradiographs, histology, and immunohistochemistry – is enormous. Original images should always be retained, and any manipulation procedures should be disclosed. The increasing use of digital images in science is one route whereby misconduct can occur. The German cancer scientists Herrman and Brach were found to have published 47 papers that contained fabricated data, one of which contained an autoradiograph, which was clearly fabricated. Many journals now insist that an electronic record of any changes made to original data outputs should be submitted with the paper.

Authorship

The International Committee of Medical Editors (the Vancouver Group) has produced guidelines on authorship that demand that each author must have contributed substantially throughout the process (Box 18.1) [13]. In the past 'gift' (or 'honorary') authorship has been employed widely. It is felt, however, that this is no longer acceptable and that the concept that the professor or head of department should inevitably find his or her way on to a paper

---

Box 18.1 Authorship (from Ref. [13])

Authorship credit should be based only on substantial contributions to:
- Conception and design or analysis and interpretation of data.
- Drafts of the article or critical revisions for important intellectual content.
- Final approval of the version to be published.

simply because the work was performed in the department is not enough to warrant authorship. Each contributor should be able to state clearly at the end of the paper how they participated in the study. Each author must take public responsibility for the work published in the paper, although, with the multidisciplinary nature of much of the work that is performed currently, it is usually advisable to have one individual, usually the senior investigator, to act as guarantor.

The three conditions of authorship must all be met. Participation solely in the acquisition of funding or the collection of data does not justify authorship. General supervision of the research group also is insufficient for authorship.

Conflicts of interest

Conflicts of interest, or competing interests, are probably more common than most of us like to admit. Competing interests can involve all participants in the publication process, including authors, reviewers, editors, and indeed the journal owners or publishers. A competing interest might be something that when revealed at some point after publication means that a reasonable reader might feel misled or deceived. The existence of competing interests is not a crime as long as they are disclosed. Reviewers also have competing interests; he or she may be a direct competitor, for example, and may wish to retard the publication of work. The journal owner or publisher may attempt to persuade editors to publish material that may be advantageous to the journal financially, at the expense of compromising scientific or academic standards. If in doubt, disclose.

Peer review

Peer review is the process used to assess the value of papers submitted to a journal with the ultimate aim of improving the quality of the paper. The conventional approach to peer review is that the authors are usually unaware of the identity of the reviewers, whereas the reviewers do know the identity of the authors. It is argued that this enables the reviewer to give a frank opinion of the work without fear of retribution. It has been considered, however, that this is an intrinsically unfair approach and, although it protects the reviewer, it may expose the author to unfair attack, particularly if the reviewer has competing scientific or other academic interests [14]. 'Open' peer review has been proposed to enhance the quality of the review, although this outcome has been hard to prove by formal evaluation. Concerns exist however that younger reviewers may be excessively exposed, particularly when commenting on the imperfections of a paper from one of the 'giants' in the field. The relationship between the author, the editor, and the peer reviewer is a confidential interaction. The manuscript should only be passed on to a colleague or other individual with the editor's permission. A reviewer or editor should not use information contained in such a paper for his or her own benefit.

Duties of editors

Editors are the custodians of the biomedical literature and have the responsibility for maintaining high standards in research and publication ethics. The editor, however, must balance the interests of the many stakeholders in the journal, including readers, authors, editorial staff including associate editors, editorial board members, the owner and/or publisher, advertisers, and the media. Competing interests may exist between stakeholders, and the editor's duty is to ensure that these do not damage the stakeholders or the journal. They should not be reluctant to publish work that challenges previously published studies in their journal, and they should not reject studies with negative results.

Recently editors have been criticised for inappropriate practices, particularly in the criteria that are used to select papers for publication. Following the retraction of papers in *Nature* and *Science* by Jan Hendrik Schon, both journals were criticised by the *Wall Street Journal*, stating that '*Nature* and *Science* are locked in such fierce competition for prestige and publicity that they may be cutting corners to get 'hot' papers'. Robert Laughlin, Nobel laureate, agreed, saying that 'in this case, the editors are definitely culpable: they chose reviewers they knew would be positive' [10]. Thus, competition between journals and their editors can result in reduction in the quality of the peer review process.

Editors must be willing to act promptly if subsequently it becomes apparent that a published paper has been published previously or contains fraudulent data. Editors should place a notice in the journal to indicate redundant publication or should formally retract the article after previously informing the authors of their intention. Retraction does not correct the paper records, however, such that retracted papers may continue to be cited without reference to their dubious content [15].

Media relations

Major medical breakthroughs now attract considerable media attention. Journalists frequently attend medical meetings where they will encounter unpublished research. It is now quite common for major discoveries to be reported in a newspaper before they appear in peer reviewed journals. Authors should be encouraged to arrange for their work to be published simultaneously in the biomedical literature and the mass media. Authors should give a balanced account of their work, drawing attention to both the strengths and weaknesses of the study. Analysis of a series of press releases has indicated that the information provided to journalists plays excessively on the strengths of the studies reported and as such tends to be unbalanced.

Research and publication misconduct

Research misconduct represents a spectrum ranging from errors of judgement (mistakes made in good faith) through what have been regarded as minor misdemeanours, so-called 'trimming and cooking' to blatant fraud, usually categorised as fabrication, falsification, and plagiarism (Box 18.2).

Box 18.2 Research misconduct

Errors of judgement
- Inadequate study design
- Bias
- Self-delusion
- Inappropriate statistical analysis

Misdemeanours ('trimming and cooking')
- Data manipulation
- Data exclusion
- Suppression of inconvenient facts

Fraud
- Fabrication
- Falsification
- Plagiarism

All stakeholders in the publishing process have the responsibility to be vigilant for possible breaches of research and publication ethics, and they should be willing to act as a 'whistleblower'. Informal surveys suggest that many investigators have suspected colleagues of research misconduct [3,16]. People are reticent about making accusations against a colleague because of the inevitable personal difficulties that might result – irrespective of whether the accusations are eventually found to be true. Information derived through this route, however, is probably the most important for exposing scientific dishonesty – it being relatively difficult to detect reliably research and publication misconduct through the peer review process. 'Whistleblowers' are usually protected by anonymity in the early stages of an investigation and, in the United Kingdom, the Public Interest Disclosure Act

1998 has provided additional legal protection for all 'whistleblowers' in the workplace. This added protection has the disadvantage that it might encourage a malcontent colleague to make false allegations behind the screen of anonymity. Experience in the United States, however, would indicate that most complaints are bona fide.

A number of published guidelines describe how institutions should investigate possible research misconduct. The Royal College of Physicians, London, has indicated that every institution should have its own system to manage complaints of scientific misconduct and has suggested a procedure as to how to take the process forward [17]. Similar guidance has been provided by the United Kingdom's Medical Research Council [18]. Other countries, such as the United States, Norway, Denmark, and other European countries, have established national agencies to deal with research integrity [19]. Currently in the United Kingdom, the GMC is responsible for considering cases for research misconduct amongst clinical investigators. Over the past few years there has been increasing interest to establish a body with a wider remit to advise on research misconduct [20–22] and this was finally achieved in May 2006 with the launch of the UK Panel for Research Integrity in Health and Biomedical Science. This now leads on research misconduct for both the university sector and the National Health Service and is producing national guidance on 'best practice' for the conduct of research and will advise on the investigation of allegations of research misconduct (www.ukrio.org.uk).

Plagiarism
Plagiarism is the use of another individual's published work or unpublished ideas without attribution. Both scientific papers and grant proposals have been used as targets for plagiarism within the field of biomedicine. The growing reservoir of electronic material and its ease of accessibility have probably facilitated the use of plagiarism to enhance authors' apparent productivity. Plagiarism may be used in some instances as a device to cover up language difficulties for those for whom English is not the first language. Authors should always be encouraged to seek help in preparing their manuscript if language is a problem and not resort to using the words of others.

Redundant publication
Redundant publication (sometimes referred to as duplicate or triplicate publication) is the term used when two or more papers that overlap in a major way are published in different journals without cross-reference [23]. If the same paper is published on two or more occasions, then the biomedical literature can become biased towards a particular hypothesis or treatment modality. This

is particularly hazardous with respect to clinical trials involving a new drug and the potential that this can have on biasing subsequent meta-analyses.

In some situations, however, it is entirely reasonable to republish already published material. Publication of an abstract as part of the proceedings of a scientific meeting does not constitute redundant publication, but full disclosure should be made when the full paper is submitted. Previous publication of a paper in another language is also acceptable, as long as it is disclosed. It is not uncommon for two or more papers involving the same or similar patient database to be published in sequence. Authors should disclose this to the editor and make cross-reference to previous papers.

Motives for misconduct?

The reasons why investigators fabricate data are not fully understood. One of the sad facts is that 'crime does seem to pay' and that fraud can remain undetected for years or even indefinitely. Pressure to produce results is often cited as a common factor, particularly when new data are required for the next grant application or an upcoming scientific meeting. There are situations when perhaps junior researchers are 'encouraged' or even coerced to 'enhance' their data by a research supervisor who has become anxious when results were not been forthcoming. Some may be enticed by financial considerations and the drive for promotion, while others may be deluded by the belief that limited preliminary experiments have 'proved the case' and that spending additional months producing confirmatory data would merely be a waste of time! The research is therefore completed on the desktop rather than in the laboratory! Whatever the reason, it is dishonest; it corrupts the scientific record and ultimately is bad for UK PLC because the commercial world will not deal with a scientific community that permits serious breaches of research conduct.

Prevention of misconduct?

The widespread nature of research and publication misconduct in all its forms and degrees of severity indicates that existing control measures are inadequate. Improved methods for the detection of misconduct are required, as is the increased vigilance of research supervisors, laboratory co-workers, and all those involved in the publication process. Even if 'policing' of research were made more effective, it would not address the fundamental issue of why some individuals advertently or inadvertently betray their responsibilities as a scientist or clinical investigator. Clear guidance on ethics should be emphasised during research training and in all institutions actively involved in research [24]. This should be accompanied, however, by endorsement of the research ethos of quality rather than quantity. A variety of other interventions may also assist (Box 18.3).

Box 18.3 Prevention of research and publication misconduct

Education
- Research training
- Research ethics
- Publication ethics

The research
- Protocol driven
- Establish contributors and collaborators
  - Define roles
  - Agree protocol
  - Agree presentation of results
- Define methodology for data analysis
  - Statistical advice
- Ethical approval
- Project and personal licence (Home Office)
- Supervision
  - Identify guarantor
  - Good communication
  - Ensure good clinical practice
- Meticulous record keeping

The publication
- Disclose conflict of interest
- Disclose previous publications
- Approval by all contributors
- Submit to one journal at a time
- Assume research data audit

A key step in the prevention of research and publication misconduct is education. Institutional guidelines should be available to all researchers as they join a new institution, and formal instruction in research and publication ethics should be part of research training and a component of all taught and non-taught courses.

Close supervision of a research project is an essential component of research integrity. Research misconduct may be more prevalent when investigators are isolated, possibly believing that 'they can get away with it because no one else will know'. Inadequate review of raw data by a project supervisor may facilitate falsification or fabrication in large prestigious departments in which young investigators feel excessive pressure to produce results. Research integrity is dependent on good communication between contributors, with frequent discussion on the progress of the project and openness about any difficulties encountered in adhering to the research protocol. Protocol changes should be agreed by all. *Good Clinical Practice* guidelines should be adhered to in all clinical studies. Record keeping must be of the highest quality. By law, case report forms from all clinical trials and other clinical studies must be kept for 15 years. Laboratory investigators must keep records of all experiments performed, which include original data printouts and any other paper or photographic record of experimental results. These should be attached to the appropriate page in a laboratory notebook. Laboratory research records should be retained in the department in which the work has been performed and should be available for review for at least 15 years.

References

1 Farthing MJG. Research misconduct. *Gut* 1997;**41**:1–2.
2 Farthing MJG. Retractions in *Gut* 10 years after publication. *Gut* 2001;**48**:285–6.
3 Lock S. Research misconduct 1974–1990: an imperfect history. In: Lock S, Wells F, Farthing M, eds., *Fraud and misconduct in biomedical research*, 3rd edn. London: BMJ Publishing Group, 2001, pp. 51–63.
4 Kintisch E. Researcher faces prison for fraud in NIH Grant applications and papers. *Science* 2005;**307**:1851.
5 Dalton R. Universities scramble to assess scope of falsified results. *Nature* 2005;**438**:7.
6 Wohn Y. Seoul National University dismisses Hwang. *Science* 2006;**311**:1695.
7 Couzin J, Unger K. Cleaning up the paper trail. *Science* 2006;**312**:38–43.
8 Giles J. Plagiarism in Cambridge physics lab prompts calls for guidelines. *Nature* 2004;**427**:3.
9 Abbott A. Prolific ecologist vows to fight Danish misconduct verdict. *Nature* 2004;**427**:381.
10 Adam D, Knight J. Publish, and be damned … *Nature* 2002;**419**:772–6.
11 White C, eds. *The COPE Report 1999*. Annual Report of the Committee on Publication Ethics. London: BMJ Books, 1999.
12 Smith R. Authorship: time for a paradigm shift? *BMJ* 1997;**314**:992.
13 International Committee of Medical Journal Editors. Uniform requirements for manuscripts submitted to biomedical journals. *Ann Intern Med* 1997;**126**:36–47.
14 Smith R. Peer review: reform or revolution? Time to open up the black box of peer review. *BMJ* 1997;**315**:759–60.
15 Budd JM, Sievert ME, Schultz TR. Phenomena of retraction. *JAMA* 1998;**280**:296–7.
16 Wilmshurst P. The code of silence. *Lancet* 1997;**349**:567–9.
17 Working Party. *Fraud and misconduct in medical research. Causes, investigation and prevention*. London: Royal College of Physicians, 1991.
18 Medical Research Council. *Policy and procedure for inquiring into allegations of scientific misconduct*. Mitcham: Aldridge Print Group, 1997.

19 Nylenna M, Andersen D, Dahlquist G, Sarvas M, Aakvaag A. Handling of scientific dishonesty in the Nordic countries. *Lancet* 1999;**354**:57–61.

20 Smith R. Misconduct in research: editors respond. *BMJ* 1997;**315**:201–2.

21 Farthing MJG. An editor's response to fraudsters. *BMJ* 1998;**316**:1729–31.

22 Farthing M, Horton R, Smith R. UK's failure to act on research misconduct. *Lancet* 2000;**356**:2030.

23 Doherty M. The misconduct of redundant publication. *Ann Rheum Dis* 1996; **55**:83–5.

24 Medical Research Council. *Good research practice.* London: MRC, 2000.

Chapter 19 **Electronic publishing**

Craig Bingham

Once upon a time

When I first began working for a medical journal in 1990, articles were always submitted on paper. The review process was carried out by mail, although the practice of faxing a copy of the paper to reviewers was becoming more common. The editing of accepted manuscripts was done by marking up the paper copy with red and blue pen. A copy of this marked up manuscript would be sent to the author for approval, and any author's changes would be transferred manually to the editorial copy. Marked up papers were then sent to typesetters, who retyped the entire manuscript to produce galley proofs – long strips of shiny white paper that we would read and mark for correction before sending them back to the typesetter. When corrected galleys were finalised, these were handed to the layout designer, who worked with a razor and glue to cut and paste galleys into pages. These pages were then sent to the filmmaker to be photographed, and from the resulting films, page proofs and ultimately printer's plates would be produced. The journal was printed, and there was no electronic version. Nobody outside some specialised academic communities had heard of the Internet, and there was no World Wide Web (although it was in October 1990 that Tim Berners-Lee first invented the term) [1].

Seventeen years later, at the same medical journal, articles are usually submitted via the journal's website as electronic documents. The review process is usually conducted online, using standard forms completed inside a web browser. Accepted manuscripts are edited and style tagged in Word, which is the word processing program used by most authors, and the edited copy is emailed to the author, who makes author's corrections in the file. The manuscript editors use Word's 'track changes' feature to check what the author has done before they electronically transfer the file to the production department. There, the Word file is imported into the page layout program, where style tags are converted into standard generalised mark up language (sgml). A large part of the page layout is automatic, and when the details have been completed and the proofs checked, the electronic file is transferred to the printer in portable document format (pdf). Colour proofs and printer's plates are generated directly from the pdf files. Meanwhile, the Internet version of the journal, in both hypertext mark up language (html) and pdf, is generated from the same sgml files used to produce the print version.

This production process is now typical of most journals.

Electronic publishing: choices and links

Electronic communications are transforming journals, and this is creating new opportunities and choices for authors.

If an Internet link is available in your home or workplace, it is easier and cheaper than ever before to submit articles to journals – wherever they might be. From the journals' perspective, the Internet means it is possible to reach new readers around the world more easily and cheaply than ever before. Although many journals maintain a national or regional focus, many others are seeking to internationalise their content and cater to a world audience. This means that everyone has more places to publish, and these places have become easier to find.

Authors can now use PubMed (http://www.ncbi.nlm.nih.gov/entrez/query.fcgi) to search for articles in their subject area, identify journals that carry that subject, review abstracts to assess the standard of work published, search out the journal's Internet site (this is often as simple as clicking on a link to the journal in PubMed), read the guidelines for submissions, and zap off a submission by the appropriate channel.

Factors that might influence your choice of journal

I shall not discuss factors such as the specialisation of the journal or its prestige value, as indicated by its 'impact factor' or some other measure, but electronic publishing has introduced some new considerations that deserve to be highlighted.

Speed of publication

Anecdotal evidence from journals that conduct their manuscript submission and peer review processes via the Internet are that these are faster than the paper-based alternatives. It is not just a matter of electronic communication being faster than post (although that in itself can save weeks in relation to an international submission); there also seems to be an immediacy about electronic communications that encourages editors, reviewers, and authors to respond more promptly than they do to faxes or letters. This may represent the greater efficiency of electronic document systems compared with paper systems. If so, the extent to which it is true will depend partly on how 'user friendly' the journal's system is, and this varies from journal to journal.

Some journals offer 'fast track' publication to authors whose articles have special importance or immediate implications for clinical care. Fast track publication can be achieved by instituting rapid review and/or by publishing the article online as soon as it is ready – ahead of the print edition. Journals with fast track procedures are highly selective about which articles are eligible for consideration, and special submission instructions are available for authors who wish to be considered.

Submission and peer review process

Many journals have adopted Internet-based manuscript submission and peer review (Box 19.1). These systems require authors to do most of the administrative data entry for their submission, which can be a little tricky or tedious, but there are advantages:

- the author receives immediate confirmation that the submission has been received;
- the author can track the manuscript's progress through the editorial system online;
- lost or delayed submissions are less common because these systems flag submissions that have not progressed within the normal time.

Once an author has made one submission to a journal, subsequent submissions require less data entry.

New publication formats

Some journals are now publishing both long and short versions of articles. Some publish articles as html and pdf files and some in formats suitable for use on personal digital assistants (palmtop computers).

Accessibility

Some journals belong to journal networks such as HighWire (http://www. highwire.org) or ScienceDirect (http://www. sciencedirect.com/), and these may increase the readership of your article by making it part of a larger database. When readers search one journal, they are led also to articles in other journals of the journal network.

Box 19.1 Systems for web-based manuscript submission and peer review

Examples
- Editorial Manager (Aries Systems) <www.editorialmanager.com>: used by Elsevier Science, Australasian Medical Publishing Company, University of Chicago Press, and others.
- BioMed Central <www.biomedcentral.com>: an open-access publisher of over 170 electronic journals.
- eJournalPress <www.ejournalpress.com>: used by Nature Publishing Group, Proceedings of the National Academy of Sciences of the United States of America, Palgrave Macmillan, and others.
- Bench>Press (Highwire Press) <www.highwire.stanford.edu>: used by BMJ Publishing Group, World Health Organization, and others.
- Manuscript Central (ScholarOne) <scholarone.com>: used by Blackwell Publishing, Taylor & Francis, Oxford Journals, and others.

Common features
- The submitting author must begin by registering with the manuscript submission system. This gives the author a username and password. This step will not need to be repeated for subsequent submissions to the same journal.
- Only the submitting author has access to the online system, unless he or she shares his username and password with co-authors (not recommended).
- Submissions are made by filling in web forms and uploading files to the journal's server. Only a standard web browser is required. File uploads can be slow, and the web forms sometimes require detailed information about co-authors, ethical approvals, suggested reviewers, and so on. The submission process can be started at one time and completed at another (the system will remember the tasks already completed).
- Usually a wide variety of files (e.g. Word documents, jpeg images, tiff images, pdfs) can be uploaded, but there are limitations (e.g. not all systems will accept Excel files) and it is wise to check the instructions for authors before proceeding.
- Image files can be sent as relatively low-resolution jpeg files to reduce the file size and upload time, but high-resolution copies of images will be required eventually if the article is accepted for publication.
- The submitting author can track the manuscript's progress through editorial and peer review by logging in to the system.
- Submission of revisions is generally much simpler than the original submission process, as much of the information required is already on the system.
- If the article is accepted for publication, hard copies of some documents (such as copyright assignment or permissions) may be required.

Even more important, some journals make the full text of their journal available free on the Internet. If they do this and they participate in PubMed's LinkOut program, any reader who finds the article on PubMed can click through to the full text. A few journals give access free from the day of publication (e.g. *MJA* and *CMAJ*); others make their archives freely available a few months after publication (e.g. *Proceedings of the National Academy of Sciences*). For authors who are keen to maximise the accessibility of their work, the journal's access policy is a matter to be considered.

Electronic manuscript preparation

In the new scheme of things, authors would do well to consider that they are no longer producing 'papers'. For most journals now, the important copy of the author's work is the electronic copy, because that is the copy that will be transformed into both electronic and printed publications. Authors can assist the efficiency of this process by taking some simple steps with their word processing documents and image files. In general, electronic documents that will work well for a publisher are simple to format and produce.

The dominance of Microsoft means that a *de facto* standard for electronic documents is the Word format – particularly Word 1997, Word 2000, and Word 2003, which are interchangeable in almost all respects.

For many years, the *Uniform requirements for the submission of manuscripts to biomedical journals* [2] has provided a standard acceptable to hundreds of medical journals for the formatting of manuscripts on paper; this standard has saved authors from needing to reformat their work for different journals. What is lacking is a similar standard for electronic manuscripts. This means that authors who submit work to several journals may have to observe a variety of different rules on how to format and present their work. (Note to the International Committee of Medical Journal Editors and/or the World Association of Medical Editors: How about developing a *Uniform Word template for the submission of manuscripts to medical journals*? – it would save a lot of bother.) Below, I give general advice that will be suitable for submissions to most journals, but authors should always check the instructions provided by each journal before finalising their submission. Some journals (e.g. *Nature*, and BioMed Central journals) supply a document template designed specifically for their journal.

Tips for preparing Word documents

1 It is worth while reviewing Word's behavioural preferences, which are set up under the Tools/Options submenu. In particular, several useful items can be found under the 'Save' options. Turn off the 'Allow fast saves' option: fast

saves sound like a good idea, but they produce bloated files that are harder to email and more likely to become corrupted, particularly if the publisher attempts to translate them out of Word. Turn on 'Always create backup copy' to automatically keep the penultimate version of your manuscript (useful if your master file is lost or damaged). Turn on 'Save AutoRecover info' to guard against losses during computer crashes – this is particularly important if you are one of those people who forgets to save work early and often.

2 Learn how to use the Word features under the Tools/Autocorrect submenu. Some people turn off all autocorrection features because they are disconcerted by Word's default behaviour of adjusting capitalisation and reformatting type on the fly, but these features save a lot of time once you tune them in to match your expectations. In particular, if you have a long word like 'hypergammaglobulinaemia' that you need to type repeatedly, turn on 'Replace text as you type' and add it to the replacement list. Define a short unique key sequence as the text to replace with the long word (e.g. replace 'hy' with 'hypergammaglobulinaemia') and you can improve your typing accuracy, while lowering the number of keystrokes required.

3 Keep formatting to a minimum. I have seen authors present articles as elaborate facsimiles of the journal that they are submitting to, complete with multi-column layout, embedded pictures, and a variety of fonts – a pity, as all this formatting work will be discarded by the journal as the first step towards making the author's file useful. It also annoys editors, who much prefer manuscripts in a simple one-column layout. Only use fonts that everybody has on their computers: for example, Times New Roman for your main text font and Arial as your font for headings. Turn off type justification, automatic hyphenation, and automatic paragraph numbering. On the other hand, the use of bold, italic, superscript, and subscript text as appropriate is good.

4 Use styles and style tagging rather than formatting the article paragraph by paragraph. This makes it much easier to format an article as you write and easier again if you are asked to change the formatting later. For your level 1 headings, therefore, define a Heading1 style, with the combination of font, spacing, and alignment that you want to use, and then apply this to each heading as you create it. To change all your level 1 headings later, simply redefine the style and all will be changed without having to select and manipulate each heading.

5 Format text as one continuous flow. Use a page break (Ctrl + Enter) to start a new page (e.g. after your title page) not a stream of hard returns. Some journals prefer you to put only one hard return between each paragraph, others prefer two, but more than two is a nuisance. Do not break the article up with Word's section breaks.

6 Do not use a string of spaces as a formatting device in tables or any-where else. Although text formatted this way may look correct on your computer, it becomes distorted once it is translated from Word into the publisher's desktop publishing system. To set text at a certain position on the page, use a tab – not a string of tabs, but one tab, defined to be in the right place (to set tabs, select 'Tabs' under the 'Format' menu, or view the ruler and drag the tabs to the right locations).

7 Keep table formatting simple and consistent. A common error is to place a column of separate items into a single table cell, with each item sepa-rated by a hard return: instead each data item should have a table cell of its own. Sometimes tables are formatted with tabs instead of cells: in this case, the key is to set the tab stops for the whole table so that one tab equals one column.

8 Most publishers ask you not to embed image files or other objects in your Word document. Most publishers' production systems will choke on this non-text material when they try to import your Word file, and images are frequently processed by people within the publisher's pro-duction team who will not be dealing with your text. Image files should be sent as separate files (other requirements of image files are discussed below). The same goes for Excel spreadsheets or charts. If you are embedding images in the file, it is probably best to do it at the end, after the text and references.

9 Be prepared to send the data used to generate graphs. Some publishers will use the data to regenerate the graphs according to their own style rules. In such a case, it helps if you send only the data that are actually shown in the graphs – not the spreadsheet with all of the data generated in the study.

10 Present the reference list as plain text at the end of the file, unless you are submitting to a journal that specifically endorses the use of Word's end-notes and footnotes. Word's endnotes and footnotes have some advan-tages in terms of automatic ordering and numbering, but they exist in a separate text flow and are easily lost or garbled during translations from Word to other formats. If you like to use endnotes to contain the refer-ence list during the drafting stages, you can convert them to plain text by saving your file in plain text format, but you will lose all formatting (including bold and italic) at the same time.

What about pdf?

Adobe's portable document format is designed to produce a file that will be viewed and printed from any computer that has the free Adobe Acrobat reader software installed. If you have the complete Acrobat program (not just the free reader), a pdf file can be created from Word or many other applications.

The chief advantage of a pdf is that you can be sure that the file you created can be viewed and printed exactly as you created it. This is not necessarily true of a Word file, which may be reformatted when it is displayed or printed from somebody else's computer. However, pdf files are not editable in the same way as word processor files. Some publishers will ask for, or even create, a pdf file of your manuscript for use during the peer review process, but a Word file will also be required for editing and production. Other publishers only want a Word file. Don't send a pdf if the publisher wants the manuscript sent in Word or any other word processor format.

Tips for preparing images

The most common error in preparing electronic images is to make them too small. Images appear on a computer screen at a resolution of 72 or 96 pixels per inch (ppi), but to achieve a similar quality of reproduction in print, an image will be printed at 300 dots per inch (dpi). An image that appears on screen as 4 in. (100 mm) wide at 72 ppi will only be 1 in. (25 mm) wide when printed at 300 dpi. When this image is printed at 4 in. wide, it will show jagged edges and tone blocks instead of smooth curves and gradual tone transitions.

No effective way exists to increase the resolution of an image beyond its original size, and if an image is reduced in size and saved, picture data is permanently lost. Image files therefore have to be created and saved at high resolution. For a colour image that is to be printed as 4×4 in., the required size is $(4 \times 300) \times (4 \times 300) = 1200 \times 1200 = 1\,440\,000$ dots. In many image formats (e.g. tagged image file format, or tiff), each dot will take eight bits (one byte) to store, so the image file will be 1.44 megabytes – enough to fill a floppy disk and 15–30 times the size of most image files viewed over the Internet.

Compression techniques can reduce the size of the image file, but again caution is required. Zip compression is safe, because it uses an algorithm that packs the data tighter without throwing any of it away. Compression during which files are saved in jpeg format, however, works by discarding picture data – the algorithm is very clever, and often quite a lot of compression can be applied without any discernible loss of picture quality. Flaws not evident when viewing the image on screen, however, may show up in a printed copy – particularly in the high-quality printed copy produced by a journal's press.

Most software allows you to select the level of compression you wish to apply when saving a file in jpeg format, and it is safest to select the option for large file size (maximum picture quality).

Publishers have varying requirements for image file formats, but tiff and jpeg are usually safe choices. For vector images (i.e. images such as graphs and charts generated by a computer drawing package, in which the data are described as lines and areas (vectors) rather than as single pixels), eps (encapsulated postscript) is the best file format to use. Whatever file format you are using, it is useful to send information about the image and how it was produced along with the electronic file.

The electronic future

Electronic publishing could be said to be the central technology of the scientific medical literature, but it is far from a mature technology. The recommendations for manuscript preparation made in this chapter may date rapidly, and the core requirements of 'computer literacy' are changing constantly. We are approaching a globalised medical literature, in which it will be increasingly easy to move from article to article, journal to journal, without interruption. Exactly how this will be paid for remains uncertain. Commercial publishers tend to look for 'pay-per-view' or subscription revenues – an Internet with regular tollbooths – while many academic institutions, governmental authorities, and some professional organisations favour hidden subsidy models in which Internet access to the literature is apparently free to the reader. Technologies and business models for both systems are developing competitively. Readers' preferences may be decisive, but authors are also influential – through their choice of where to submit articles for publication.

References

1 W3C. *A Little History of the World Wide Web*. Available from http://www.w3.org/History.html (accessed 2 March 2007).
2 International committee of medical journal editors. Uniform requirements for manuscripts submitted to biomedical journals. http://www.icmje.org (accessed 2 March 2007).

Chapter 20 **Open access**

Mark Ware

What is open access?

Put simply, open access is the idea of providing unrestricted online access to scholarly literature, so that anyone can make use of it without having to pay for a subscription, site licence, or per-article fee [1].

To expand a little, to qualify as fully open access the material needs to be freely available online:
- without payment or access barriers such as registration,
- immediately on publication,
- in perpetuity,
- without restrictions on its (reasonable) reuse.

Open access is an attribute of individual articles, not necessarily the journal. Journals can, and do, contain a mixture of open access and restricted material.

Making an article open access is not the same as putting it into the public domain, which involves the author giving up all rights over how the material is used. By contrast, with open access the author usually *retains* the copyright but grants a set of rights to anyone wishing to make use of it. Under the licence most commonly used for open access academic papers, users are permitted to download and save a copy, print it, read it, circulate copies, use it for teaching or research, in fact more or less anything a scientist or clinician might want to do, except that she *may not* make any commercial reuse and *must* attribute the original author. Instead of 'All rights reserved', for open access it is a case of 'Some rights reserved'.

Open access is particularly relevant for authors who want their work to be widely read, circulated, cited, debated, and built upon. It is thus a good match for the authors of journal articles, who are not seeking direct financial reward from the sale of their work (unlike a book author, say).

Why should I care about open access?

There are three main reasons:
1 You believe it will benefit you, through the greater visibility and use of your work, leading to more citations and increased reputation.
2 You believe it will benefit others and/or society at large.
3 You are required by your research funder or employer to deposit your articles in an open access repository.
We shall discuss these in more detail below.

How do I make my articles open access?

There are two main ways of making an article open access: open access *publication* (sometimes known as the 'Gold' route) and deposit by the author in an open online repository (the 'Green' route, also called *self-archiving*).

Open access publications
Open access journals do not rely on subscriptions or other kinds of payments by readers or their libraries for their income, and can thus make their content freely available.

Instead, one of the revenue sources is to levy a per-article publication charge. Article charges typically range from $1000 to $3000. Journals with publication charges usually have arrangements to reduce or eliminate these charges for authors unable to afford them (e.g. those from less developed countries).

By no means all open access journals, however, levy publication charges. Perhaps surprisingly, a slight majority have no such charges. They rely instead on a variety of funding streams such as grants, sponsorship, advertising, subscription to the print edition, support by the host institution, and so on.

The Directory of Open Access Journals (DOAJ) lists (in February 2007) about 2560 journals which can be searched or browsed by subject category [2].

Hybrid and partially open access journals
In addition to fully open access journals, there is a large number of journals offering hybrid or partial open access. The main variants are:
• *Optional open access*: Subscription journals that will allow authors (in return for a publication charge, similar in size to that charged by fully open access journals) to make their individual articles open access. This is probably the most numerous type of open access *journal*. Take-up by authors has been, however, low to date (e.g. 3–11% of authors took up this option in a recent OUP trial, and many other journals have no uptake at all as yet), so this currently represents a small fraction of open access *articles*.

- *Delayed open access*: Subscription journals that make their content open access after a set period (anything from 2 to 24 or more months). There are some 1.6 million such DOA articles hosted on HighWire alone, making this the most popular kind of open access by article numbers.
- *Hybrid journals*: These offer open access to some kinds of content, typically research articles, while still requiring a subscription to access the other types of content (e.g. review articles or journalistic content).

Self-archiving

The other route to open access is for authors to deposit a copy of their journal articles in an open repository.

There are two kinds of repository. *Subject-based repositories* offer a centralised resource for a particular discipline. *Institutional repositories* host the outputs (not just research) of a particular body, such as a university. In theory, it should not matter much which an author chooses, because the repository software is designed to support interoperability, allowing all repositories to be searched through a single search interface. In practice, researchers in a particular field may be accustomed to using a well-known repository (such as PubMed) but be unaware of ways to find content from institutional repositories; and secondly, a centralised service like PubMed can impose discipline on the metadata (such as keywords or subject headings) used to describe articles, permitting a more effective search interface. Improvements in, and more widespread use of, services like Google Scholar and Microsoft's Academic Live search will tend to negate these advantages.

Authors frequently worry that deposit in a repository will contravene the assignment of copyright they have made to the journal publisher. Perhaps surprisingly, this is often not the case – the majority of publishers and journals permit authors to archive some version of the article. Typically this version is the *post-print*, that is, the final draft following refereeing but prior to copy-editing by the publisher.

Many journals also attach some conditions to self-archiving. Many will require an embargo period between publication and the earliest the article can be made open access. Others will require a URL linking to the official version on the publisher's website.

Publishers' policies with regard to self-archiving can be conveniently checked at the RoMEO website [3].

Arguments in favour of open access

We have seen a little of how making an article open access might benefit you as an author by gaining a wider audience, perhaps leading to more citations, thereby increasing your reputation and attracting new research partners.

Let's now step back and look at some broader arguments in favour of open access [4].

First, it is argued that open access gives greater visibility and accessibility to the literature, and thus leads to greater impact from research. There is evidence that open access increases impact by substantially increasing the number of times an article is downloaded and cited. There is though some debate on the extent to which these increases are due to the open access status compared to other factors (such as authors preferentially archiving their better work).

Secondly, open access may promote the more rapid and efficient progress of research. For instance, research has shown that over the last 15 years, the period between articles being deposited in an open repository and their being cited has shortened considerably.

Thirdly, open access could facilitate the better assessment, monitoring, and management of science. Bibliometric tools that allow the study of the web of citations within a field have existed for some time, but it is argued that such tools would be much more effective if all the scientific literature were open to them.

Fourthly, novel information can be created using new computational technologies (e.g. data- and text-mining). These technologies are currently in their infancy but are already showing some promise. Although this can be done in theory with paid for content, it would be easier and more effective if the literature were transparently open to the software tools.

Fifthly, it is argued that open access journals offer greater economic efficiency than subscription-based journals. When the marginal cost of supplying another electronic copy of an article approaches zero, it is more efficient not to charge for access, because any price, however low, deters some potential users.

Lastly, it is felt by many (particularly in the United States) that the public should have the right to access outputs of research that was funded by the taxpayer. Not only is this an argument of equity, but it is also bolstered by the argument that society as a whole is better off.

Arguments against open access

The benefits of open access are, however, not uncontested.

First, some are sceptical as to whether the available business models for open access journals are sustainable or achievable. A related criticism of the publication charge model is that a widespread move to it from the present subscription model would require large and impractical shifts of funding within academia.

It may be said that this does not matter, because the market will sort it out, but critics say that it is irresponsible to promote a move from a working system to an unproven model.

Turning to the self-archiving option, critics charge that it is parasitic on the existing subscription journals. Authors still want to be published in reputable and relevant journals. If funding bodies then require them to archive their articles, the concern is that when the level of archiving reaches some critical point, libraries will abandon their paid subscriptions in favour of the free versions.

Proponents of self-archiving say this fear is unfounded because evidence from physics shows that journals can co-exist with archives even when the latter contain the same articles, or that if subscription journals do become unsustainable the transition will be manageable.

It has been said that article publication charges may discriminate against those without research funding, or at poorer institutions, or in poorer countries. Most if not all open access journals, however, offer reduced rates or free publication to such authors.

Another criticism is that open access journals may have a financial incentive to accept poor quality work, because the more articles are published, the more publication charges are levied. In fact, subscription journals face the same temptation because bigger journals sell for higher subscription prices. In practice, good journals of either persuasion depend crucially on the quality of their published content to attract authors and readers, and will isolate their peer review and editorial decision-making processes from the business side of the journal.

Self-archiving does raise some concerns about the proliferation of different versions of the same article. The post-print should not differ materially (in its scientific content) from the final publisher's version but the copy-editing process will have introduced some changes, and in some cases these could be important.

Research funders' policies

Research funders have recently started to introduce policies requesting or requiring researchers funded by them to deposit published articles resulting from the funded research in open archives.

There is a mixture of reasons for this but essentially the funders appear to have accepted the argument that they will get greater value from their investments in research the more widely the results are disseminated.

These policies are increasingly becoming mandatory, because experience shows that when deposit is voluntary, the proportion of authors choosing to self-archive is small (around 4–15%). Surveys of authors, by contrast, have shown that around 95% say they will deposit if required to do so by an employer or funder.

The funders' policies vary in five main ways: whether deposit is voluntary (but encouraged) or compulsory; which version of the article must be deposited (typically it is the post-print); the maximum delay after publication before the article is freely available (if specified, this is typically either 6 or 12 months; an alternative formulation is 'as soon as possible while complying with the publisher's policies'); whether or not they will fund open access publication charges; and the place of deposit (NIH and Wellcome specify PubMed Central and UK PubMed Central, respectively; other funders allow the author to select an appropriate subject or institutional repository).

If you have been funded by a body with a deposit policy in force, the requirements will have already been communicated to you. You can if you wish, however, look up the policies of research funders on at least two websites, ROARMAP or (probably preferable for most readers of this book) JULIET [5].

References and further information

1 Open Access Overview, by Peter Suber, provides a good introduction to the subject. http://www.earlham.edu/~peters/fos/overview.htm. There are also links on Suber's website to lots of further reading.
2 The Directory of Open Access Journals (DOAJ) lists over 2560 journals, searchable or browseable by subject area. http://www.doaj.org/
3 ROMEO – this website maintains a database of publisher policies regarding self-archiving. http://www.sherpa.ac.uk/projects/sherparomeo.html
4 This section draws on Alma Swan's excellent article Open Access: why should we have it? Cahiers de Documentation/Bladen voor Documentatie, 2006/4 (December 2006).
5 JULIET – an online database of research funder policies on research self-archiving. http://www.sherpa.ac.uk/juliet/. ROARMAP (http://www.eprints.org/openaccess/policysignup/) has similar information and also includes university policies.

Index